Student Success in Anatomy – SBAs and EMQs

Student Success in Anatomy – SBAs and EMQs

HELEN BUTLER
BA (Hons) (Oxon), MBBS, DRCOG
Foundation Year One Doctor,
The Princess Alexandra Hospital NHS Trust
North East Thames Foundation School

Edited by

NEEL SHARMA
BSc (Hons), MBChB, MSc
Core Medical Trainee Year One,
Lewisham Healthcare NHS Trust
and Honorary Clinical Lecturer in Medical Education,
Barts and the London School of Medicine and Dentistry

Foreword by

THIAGO VILLANUEVA
General Practitioner
Former BMJ Clegg Scholar
Past Editor of the Student BMJ

Radcliffe Publishing
London • New York

Radcliffe Publishing Ltd
33–41 Dallington Street
London
EC1V 0BB
United Kingdom

www.radcliffepublishing.com

Electronic catalogue and worldwide online ordering facility.

British Library Cataloguing in Publication Data
A catalogue record for this book is available from the British Library.

ISBN-13: 978 184619 508 2

The paper used for the text pages of this book
is FSC® certified. FSC (The Forest Stewardship
Council®) is an international network to promote
responsible management of the world's forests.

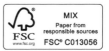

Typeset by Darkriver Design, Auckland, New Zealand
Printed and bound by TJI Digital, Padstow, Cornwall, UK

Contents

Foreword

Clinical anatomy is probably the flagship of subjects taught during medical school, and thus it might be worth taking the time to learn it well. The good news is that, when taught beyond the pure standard descriptive approach, it can actually end up catering for some tolerable, and even fun, learning. In this latest educational venture, Dr Helen Butler and Dr Neel Sharma have definitely done their homework. Not only does this book have lots of descriptive detail, always handy to gain a quick overview or engage in some last-minute reviewing, but it also has clinical pearls that help improve understanding of these often complex issues and foster effective and entertaining learning. In addition, the extensive use of mnemonics is invaluable, not only in exam situations but also when examining patients. This SBA and EMQ book goes well out of its way in helping you to plough through the nitty-gritty of anatomy in preparation for exams. In my view, it also has the potential to appeal to trainees and senior doctors for reviewing purposes, since clinical anatomy is something that takes a long time to learn, but is something that can be so easily forgotten.

Dr Tiago Villanueva
General Practitioner
Former BMJ Clegg Scholar
Past Editor of the *Student BMJ*
September 2011

Preface

As recent medical graduates we understand all too well the pressures faced during medical school. Lectures, tutorials, never-ending ward rounds, outpatient clinics, course work assignments and, of course, let us not forget the gruelling end-of-year exams. Trying to retain and, more importantly, understand all the common (and not-so-common) clinical diseases and basic science truly seems an impossible task.

This self-assessment book is designed to help students tackle questions covering all commonly tested aspects of anatomy; questions are included as SBA and EMQ formats with relevant, concise explanations as answers.

We sincerely hope that this book is of use in preparing for your forthcoming examinations and we wish you all the success in your future medical careers.

Helen Butler
Neel Sharma
September 2011

About the author

Helen Butler completed her preclinical training at Oxford University, gaining a degree in medical sciences in 2007. She then graduated from Barts and the London School of Medicine and Dentistry in 2010 with Distinctions in Clinical Science and Clinical Practice.

Helen is currently working as a Foundation Year One Doctor at The Princess Alexandra Hospital NHS Trust. She will continue her training on the Academic Foundation Programme in the North West Thames Foundation School and hopes to pursue a career in academic medicine.

About the editor

Neel Sharma graduated from Manchester University School of Medicine in 2007. He completed his foundation training in North East Thames and subsequently undertook a Master's degree in Gastroenterology.

Neel has a strong interest in medical education, having authored and edited textbooks at both undergraduate and postgraduate levels. He is currently a core medical trainee at Lewisham Healthcare NHS Trust and has been appointed as Honorary Clinical Lecturer in Medical Education at Barts and the London School of Medicine and Dentistry.

Education and work are the levers to uplift a people. Work alone will not do it unless inspired by the right ideals and guided by intelligence.

WEB Du Bois, 1868–1963

I dedicate this book to my Mum and Dad. Thank you for all your love and support, and for the sacrifices you have made to get me to where I am today.

HELEN BUTLER

I would like to dedicate this book to my parents, Ravi and Anita, and my sister Ravnita. Without their continued support and encouragement none of this would have truly been possible.

NEEL SHARMA

Questions

Section 1: Neuroanatomy

Single best answer

1 Which spinal tract carries the sensory modalities of pain and temperature?

  a Spinocerebellar tract

  b Corticospinal tract

  c Rubrospinal tract

  d Spinothalamic tract

  e Fasciculus gracilis

2 Through which structure does the olfactory nerve pass?

  a Superior orbital fissure

  b Hypoglossal canal

  c Jugular foramen

  d Stylomastoid foramen

  e Cribriform plate

3 Which of the following nerves innervate taste to the posterior third of the tongue?

   a Glossopharyngeal nerve

   b Hypoglossal nerve

   c Facial nerve

   d Vagus nerve

   e Mandibular branch of the trigeminal nerve

4 At which intervertebral level does the spinal cord terminate in adult life?

   a L1–L2

   b T11–T12

   c S2–S3

   d L5–S1

   e S3–S4

5 Through which cranial layer does the middle meningeal artery pass?

   a Extradural

   b Subdural

   c Subarachnoid

   d Cisterna magna

   e Beneath the pia mater

6 Which structure of the middle ear is supplied by the facial nerve?

a Stapedius

b Tympanic membrane

c Malleus

d Eustachian tube

e External auditory meatus

7 Which of the following arteries supply the occipital lobe?

a Anterior cerebral artery

b Middle cerebral artery

c Posterior cerebral artery

d Basilar artery

e Anterior communicating artery

8 From which structure is oxytocin secreted?

a Adrenal gland

b Posterior pituitary gland

c Parathyroid gland

d Anterior pituitary gland

e Pineal gland

9 Which of the following nerves innervate the afferent limb of the corneal reflex?

a Oculomotor nerve

b Trochlear nerve

c Ophthalmic branch of the trigeminal nerve

d Facial nerve

e Abducens nerve

10 Which of the following lesions would result in unilateral facial weakness with sparing of the forehead?

a Facial nerve: upper motor neuron lesion

b Facial nerve: lower motor neuron lesion

c Trigeminal nerve: lesion of the mandibular branch

d Glossopharyngeal nerve lesion

e Trigeminal nerve: lesion of the maxillary branch

11 Through which structure does the maxillary branch of the trigeminal nerve pass?

a Foramen rotundum

b Foramen spinosum

c Foramen lacerum

d Foramen ovale

e Superior orbital fissure

12 Which of the following nerves is responsible for lateral gaze?

a Abducens nerve

b Trochlear nerve

c Oculomotor nerve

d Optic nerve

e Facial nerve

13 Which of the following arteries supply the frontal and medial cerebrum?

a Posterior cerebral artery

b Anterior cerebral artery

c Middle cerebral artery

d Posterior inferior cerebellar artery

e Anterior spinal artery

14 Which structure runs in the subdural space?

a Middle meningeal artery

b Dural veins

c Internal jugular vein

d Trabecula

e Internal carotid artery

15 The following are all components of the basal ganglia EXCEPT:

a Globus pallidus

b Caudate nucleus

c Mammillary bodies

d Striatum

e Putamen

16 Which of the following results in a bitemporal hemianopia?

a Parietal lobe infarct

b Occipital lobe infarct

c Optic nerve lesion

d Optic chiasm compression

e Temporal lobe infarct

17 Which extraocular muscle is supplied by the trochlear nerve?

  a Inferior oblique

  b Superior oblique

  c Lateral rectus

  d Medial rectus

  e Superior rectus

18 Deviation of the tongue towards the left on protrusion indicates a lesion to which of the following structures?

  a Left glossopharyngeal nerve

  b Left facial nerve

  c Right glossopharyngeal nerve

  d Left hypoglossal nerve

  e Right hypoglossal nerve

19 Which of the following nerves pass through the foramen rotundum?

  a Ophthalmic branch of the trigeminal nerve

  b Mandibular branch of the trigeminal nerve

  c Maxillary branch of the trigeminal nerve

  d Glossopharyngeal nerve

  e Facial nerve

20 Which of the following structures traverse the foramen ovale?

a Maxillary branch of the trigeminal nerve

b Mandibular branch of the trigeminal nerve

c Internal carotid artery

d Facial nerve

e Ophthalmic artery

21 From which vessel does the ophthalmic artery branch?

a Internal carotid artery

b Vertebral artery

c External carotid artery

d Basilar artery

e Posterior inferior cerebellar artery

22 Which of the following structures correspond to the point at which the dorsal columns decussate?

a Medulla

b Pons

c Midbrain

d Ventral white commissure

e Somatosensory cortex

23 Which structure is responsible for the formation of cerebrospinal fluid?

    a Pia mater

    b Choroid plexus

    c Cisterna magna

    d Dural venous sinuses

    e Tentorium cerebelli

24 Where is the primary somatosensory cortex located?

    a Occipital lobe

    b Frontal lobe

    c Temporal lobe

    d Parietal lobe

    e Cerebellum

25 Which cells are responsible for the production of the myelin sheath?

    a Pacinian corpuscles

    b Microglia

    c Merkel's disks

    d Oligodendrocytes

    e Astrocytes

26 The following are all signs of a lower motor neuron lesion EXCEPT:

a Wasting

b Hypotonia

c Hyperreflexia

d Weakness

e Fasciculations

27 Which of the following is secreted from the posterior pituitary gland?

a Gonadotrophin-releasing hormone

b Prolactin

c Antidiuretic hormone

d Follicle-stimulating hormone

e Thyroid-stimulating hormone

28 The precentral gyrus is also known as which of the following?

a Primary somatosensory cortex

b Primary visual cortex

c Primary motor cortex

d Wernicke's area

e Broca's area

29 Which of the following causes a subacute combined degeneration of the cord?

a Lyme disease

b Multiple sclerosis

c Guillain–Barré syndrome

d Vitamin B_{12} deficiency

e Alcohol abuse

30 Which visual defect would you expect in a right-sided temporal lobe infarct?

a Left-sided homonymous hemianopia

b Right-sided superior quadrantanopia

c Left-sided inferior quadrantanopia

d Left-sided superior quadrantanopia

e Bitemporal hemianopia

31 Which of the following is NOT a branch of the facial nerve?

a Cervical branch

b Temporal branch

c Zygomatic branch

d Maxillary branch

e Buccal branch

32 Which of the following is an area in the inferior frontal gyrus that is responsible for speech?

   a Wernicke's area

   b Broca's area

   c Articulation area

   d Precentral gyrus

   e Cingulate gyrus

33 Charcot's triad comprises which three signs?

   a Resting tremor, ataxia, dysarthria

   b Wide-based gait, dyskinesia, intention tremor

   c Rigidity, dyskinesia, resting tremor

   d Nystagmus, rigidity, dysarthria

   e Dysarthria, nystagmus, intention tremor

34 A 73-year-old man presents to his GP with a festinant gait, a resting 'pill-rolling' tremor and generalised rigidity. Which of the following is true with regard to his condition?

   a Deletion of the dystrophin gene on the X chromosome

   b Loss of dopaminergic neurons in the nigrostriatal pathway

   c Loss of neurons in the hippocampal formation

   d Loss of gamma-aminobutyric acid (GABA)ergic neurons in the striatum

   e None of the above

35 Which of the following structures is associated with the nerve supplying shoulder elevation?

a Internal acoustic meatus

b Superior orbital fissure

c Jugular foramen

d Optic canal

e Foramen magnum

36 Through which structure does cerebrospinal fluid drain from the third ventricle before passing into the fourth ventricle?

a Lateral ventricle

b Interventricular foramen

c Foramen of Luschka

d Foramen of Magendie

e Cerebral aqueduct

37 Which neurological disorder is characterised by the triad of ophthalmoplegia, ataxia and confusion?

a Korsakoff's syndrome

b Normal pressure hydrocephalus

c Wernicke's encephalopathy

d Alzheimer's disease

e Pick's disease

38 Which foramen, located directly beneath the posterior clinoid process, allows the passage of the internal carotid artery?

a Foramen rotundum

b Foramen ovale

c Foramen spinosum

d Foramen lacerum

e Jugular foramen

39 Which structure does NOT pass through the foramen magnum?

a Medulla oblongata

b Vertebral arteries

c Spinal root of the accessory nerve

d Facial nerve

e Cerebellar tonsils

40 Where is the primary visual cortex located?

a Calcarine sulcus

b Precentral gyrus

c Broca's area

d Parieto-occipital sulcus

e Postcentral gyrus

Extended matching questions

Theme: Where is the lesion?

    a Optic chiasm

    b Parietal lobe

    c Temporal lobe

    d Frontal lobe

    e Occipital lobe

    f Right optic nerve

    g Left optic nerve

    h Right oculomotor nerve

    i Left oculomotor nerve

    j Abducens nerve

    k Trochlear nerve

For each of the following scenarios described, select the most appropriate answer from the above list of options. Each option may be used once, more than once or not at all.

1 Visual field examination demonstrating a superior quadrantanopia.

2 A man presenting with 'tunnel vision' and found on examination to have a bitemporal hemianopia.

3 A 33-year-old woman complaining of double vision. On examination she is unable to abduct her left eye.

4 On shining a light into the right eye, the left pupil constricts, while the right does not.

5 A 78-year-old man in the stroke unit with an inferior quadrantanopia.

Theme: Anatomy of the cranial foramina

a Foramen ovale

b Foramen rotundum

c Foramen spinosum

d Superior orbital fissure

e Foramen lacerum

f Cribriform plate

g Optic canal

h Stylohyoid foramen

i Jugular foramen

For each of the following questions, select the most appropriate answer from the above list of options. Each option may be used once, more than once or not at all.

1   Through which foramen does the olfactory nerve pass?

2   Through which foramen does the maxillary branch of the trigeminal pass?

3   Through which foramen does the facial nerve pass?

4   Through which foramen does the trochlear nerve pass?

5   Through which foramen does the mandibular branch of cranial nerve V pass?

Theme: Neuroendocrinology

a Parathyroid gland

b Medial preoptic nucleus

c Anterior pituitary gland

d Posterior pituitary gland

e Adrenal gland

f Caudate nucleus

g Nucleus accumbens

h Suprachiasmatic nucleus

i Arcuate nucleus

For each of the following questions, select the most appropriate answer from the above list of options. Each option may be used once, more than once or not at all.

1 Which structure is responsible for oxytocin secretion?

2 Which structure is responsible for maintaining circadian rhythm?

3 Which structure is responsible for maintaining thyroid function?

4 Which structure forms part of the striatum?

5 Which structure is responsible for the secretion of adrenocortico-trophic hormone?

Theme: Anatomy of the spinal tracts

a Spinocerebellar tract

b Optic tract

c Corticospinal tract

d Spinothalamic tract

e Thalamocortical tract

f Internal capsule

g Sympathetic trunk

h Dorsal columns

For each of the following questions, select the most appropriate answer from the above list of options. Each option may be used once, more than once or not at all.

1 Which tract passes between the putamen and caudate of the basal ganglia?

2 Which tract is responsible for carrying sensory information relating to pain and temperature?

3 Which tract runs from the optic chiasm to the lateral geniculate nucleus?

4 Which tract is a descending motor tract?

5 Which tract decussates as the medial lemniscus?

Theme: Anatomy of the cranial nerves

a Trigeminal nerve

b Facial nerve

c Abducens nerve

d Accessory nerve

e Hypoglossal nerve

f Oculomotor nerve

g Olfactory nerve

h Optic nerve

i Trochlear nerve

j Vestibulocochlear nerve

k Glossopharyngeal nerve

l Vagus nerve

For each of the following questions, select the most appropriate answer from the above list of options. Each option may be used once, more than once or not at all.

1 Which nerve provides motor function to the muscles of mastication?

2 Which nerve provides taste sensation to the anterior two-thirds of the tongue?

3 Which nerve provides the efferent limb of the pupillary light reflex?

4 Which nerve innervates the sternocleidomastoid muscle?

5 Which nerve provides the afferent limb of the corneal reflex upon tactile stimulation of the cornea?

Section 2: Musculoskeletal system

Single best answer

1   A 29-year-old man is rushed to the Accident and Emergency department following a roadtraffic accident. He complains of pain in his right shoulder and an X-ray demonstrates evidence of an anterior dislocation. Neurological examination reveals loss of sensation over the 'regimental badge' area of his right arm. Which nerve is most likely to have been damaged?

a   Radial nerve

b   C3–C4

c   Medial nerve

d   Axillary nerve

e   Suprascapular nerve

2   Which of the following best describes the point midway between the anterior superior iliac spine and the pubic tubercle?

   a   The position of the femoral artery

   b   The position of the superficial inguinal ring

   c   The position of the deep inguinal ring

   d   The mid-inguinal point

   e   McBurney's point

3   Which of the following nerves innervate the serratus anterior?

   a   Dorsal scapular nerve

   b   Long thoracic nerve

   c   Suprascapular nerve

   d   Axillary nerve

   e   Musculocutaneous nerve

4   Which of the following is NOT a muscle of the rotator cuff?

   a   Subscapularis

   b   Teres major

   c   Teres minor

   d   Infraspinatus

   e   Supraspinatus

5 Which of the following pulses can be palpated posterior to the medial malleolus?

a Popliteal pulse

b Femoral pulse

c Posterior tibial

d Anterior tibial

e Dorsalis pedis

6 Which tendon facilitates flexion of the distal interphalangeal joint of the index finger?

a Flexor digitorum profundus

b Flexor digitorum superficialis

c Flexor pollicis brevis

d Flexor digiti minimi brevis

e Palmar interossei

7 The median nerve innervates all of the following muscles EXCEPT:

a Adductor pollicis brevis

b Abductor pollicis brevis

c Flexor pollicis brevis

d Quadratus

e Opponens pollicis

8   Which three structures form the boundaries of the femoral triangle?

   a   Sartorius, gluteus maximus, psoas major

   b   Iliacus, sartorius, pectineus

   c   Sartorius, rectus femoris, inguinal ligament

   d   Adductor longus, inguinal ligament, sartorius

   e   Rectus femoris, gracilis, sartorius

9   Which structure lies immediately lateral to the femoral artery?

   a   Femoral nerve

   b   Femoral vein

   c   Deep inguinal lymph nodes

   d   Superficial inguinal ring

   e   Pubic tubercle

10   Which of the following nerves provide sensation to the lateral three and a half digits of the hand?

   a   Median nerve

   b   Ulnar nerve

   c   Radial nerve

   d   Musculocutaneous nerve

   e   Axillary nerve

11 Which nerve innervates the hamstring muscles?

   a T12–L1

   b Internal iliac nerve

   c External iliac nerve

   d Sciatic nerve

   e Femoral nerve

12 Which of the following nerves traverse the carpal tunnel and can be damaged by compression of this area?

   a Ulnar nerve

   b Axillary nerve

   c Medial nerve

   d Radial nerve

   e Musculoskeletal nerve

13 Which of the following is a branch of the internal iliac artery?

   a Superior mesenteric artery

   b Femoral artery

   c Popliteal artery

   d Posterior tibial artery

   e Superior gluteal artery

14 Which of the following arteries can be palpated in the antecubital fossa?

a   Radial artery

b   Median artery

c   Ulnar artery

d   Brachial artery

e   Axillary artery

15 Which bone sits in the glenoid fossa?

a   Femur

b   Humerus

c   Radius

d   Tibia

e   Fibula

16 Which of the following arteries supply the anterior compartment of the lower leg?

a   Deep femoral artery

b   Posterior tibial artery

c   Anterior tibial artery

d   Peroneal artery

e   Popliteal artery

17 Which of the following is responsible for dorsiflexion of the ankle?

a Tibialis anterior

b Gastrocnemius

c Soleus

d Flexor digitorum longus

e Tibialis posterior

18 Which of the following is an example of a sesamoid bone?

a Fibula

b Triquetral

c Patella

d Tibia

e Calcaneum

19 Which of the following is NOT a ligament of the knee joint?

a Anterior cruciate

b Medial collateral

c Lateral collateral

d Posterior cruciate

e Anterior collateral

20 Which nerve supplies the latissimus dorsi?

a Long thoracic nerve

b Musculocutaneous nerve

c Axillary nerve

d Suprascapular nerve

e Thoracodorsal nerve

21 Which structure connects adjacent spinal laminae?

a Ligamentum flava

b Interspinous ligaments

c Ligamentum arteriosum

d Longitudinal ligaments

e Ligamentum nuchae

22 Which muscle facilitates sitting cross-legged?

a Sartorius

b Gluteus maximus

c Biceps femoris

d Popliteus

e Gracilis

23 Which of the following is NOT a member of the quadriceps muscle group?

a Vastus medialis

b Vastus intermedius

c Vastus lateralis

d Semitendinosus

e Rectus femoris

24 Which of the following nerves innervate the quadriceps?

a Sciatic nerve

b Tibial nerve

c Femoral nerve

d Obturator nerve

e Deep peroneal nerve

25 Which of the following is a branch of the internal carotid artery?

a Inferior hypophyseal artery

b Ophthalmic artery

c Central artery of the retina

d Middle cerebral artery

e All of the above

26 Which of the following is responsible for opening of the mouth?

a Masseter

b Temporalis

c Lateral pterygoid

d Medial pterygoid

e All of the above

27 The dorsalis pedis originates from which of the following arteries?

a Anterior tibial artery

b Posterior tibial artery

c Peroneal artery

d Internal iliac artery

e Deep femoral artery (deep artery of the thigh)

28 The spermatic cord forms which vestigial structure in women?

a Meckel's diverticulum

b Ductus venosus

c Round ligament

d Uterine artery

e Fallopian tube

29 Which of the following is the distal attachment of the patella tendon?

a Patella

b Tibial tuberosity

c Talus

d Fibula

e Tibia

30 Which nerve root supplies the biceps-jerk reflex?

a C3

b T3

c T1

d C5

e C7

31 Which nerve is most commonly damaged in dislocation of the hip?

a Posterior tibial nerve

b Sural nerve

c Sciatic nerve

d Femoral nerve

e S3

32 The brachial plexus is formed from the C4–T1 roots. It divides into upper, middle and lower trunks, then lateral, posterior and medial cords. Which of the following nerves arise from the lateral cord?

  a Ulnar nerve

  b Musculocutaneous nerve

  c Axillary nerve

  d Radial nerve

  e Long thoracic nerve

33 A positive Babinski (plantar) reflex indicates which of the following?

  a Ruptured Achilles tendon

  b Upper motor neuron lesion

  c Lower motor neuron lesion

  d Fractured base of the fifth metatarsal

  e Common peroneal nerve lesion

34 Which vertebra is known as the 'atlas vertebra'?

  a C1

  b C2

  c C3

  d C4

  e C5

35 Which is a common site for a Baker's cyst?

a Suprapatellar bursa

b Iliac fossa

c Antecubital fossa

d Popliteal fossa

e Glenoid fossa

36 Which nerve supplies the cricothyroid muscle?

a Recurrent laryngeal nerve

b Superior laryngeal nerve

c Internal laryngeal nerve

d Vestibulocochlear nerve

e Facial nerve

37 Tenderness in the 'anatomical snuffbox' is caused by a fracture of which bone?

a Lunate

b Hypothenar eminence

c Radius

d Ulnar

e Scaphoid

38 Which structure runs through the 'anatomical snuffbox'?

a Ulnar artery

b Radial artery

c Median artery

d Median nerve

e Ulnar nerve

39 Which vertebra has the odontoid peg?

   a C1

   b C2

   c C6

   d T1

   e T4

40 Which of the following is NOT a feature of the knee joint?

   a Bursae

   b Collateral ligaments

   c Menisci

   d Ball-and-socket joint

   e Hinge joint

Extended matching questions

Theme: Anatomy of the hand

    a Extensor digitorum

    b Opponens pollicis

    c Flexor pollicis brevis

    d Abductor pollicis brevis

    e Adductor pollicis brevis

    f Flexor digitorum superficialis

    g Flexor digitorum profundus

    h Brachial nerve

    i Ulnar nerve

    j Radial nerve

    k Median nerve

For each of the following questions, select the most appropriate answer from the above list of options. Each option may be used once, more than once or not at all.

1 Which tendon facilitates flexion of the distal interphalangeal joint?

2 Which nerve provides sensation to the lateral three and a half digits?

3 Which muscle of the thenar eminence is supplied by the ulnar nerve?

4 Which nerve provides sensation to the first web space on the dorsum of the hand?

5 Which nerve innervates the opponens pollicis?

Theme: Blood supply of the upper limbs

a Axillary artery

b Internal carotid artery

c Radial artery

d Ulnar artery

e Brachial artery

f Brachiocephalic artery

g Subclavian artery

h Basilic vein

i Cephalic vein

j Superior vena cava

k Internal jugular vein

l Subclavian vein

For each of the following questions, select the most appropriate answer from the above list of options. Each option may be used once, more than once or not at all.

1 Which artery arises from the aortic arch to supply the left upper limb?

2 From which vessel does the right subclavian artery arise?

3 Upon entering the base of the neck the axillary veins become which vessel?

4 Which artery can be palpated at the front medial aspect of the elbow?

5 Which vein drains the radial side of the forearm?

Theme: Blood supply of the lower limbs

a Valves

b Deep inguinal lymph nodes

c Short saphenous vein

d Long saphenous vein

e Dorsalis pedis artery

f Posterior tibial artery

g Peroneal artery

h Femoral artery

i Femoral vein

j Femoral nerve

For each of the following questions, select the most appropriate answer from the above list of options. Each option may be used once, more than once or not at all.

1 Which feature of the lower-limb veins helps to minimise hydrostatic pressure upon standing?

2 The femoral artery passes medial to which structure?

3 Which artery can be palpated behind the medial malleolus?

4 Which artery supplies the lateral component of the leg?

5 Which vein runs medially to drain the lower limb?

Theme: Anatomy of the upper limb

a Axillary nerve

b Ulnar nerve

c Radial nerve

d Median nerve

e Triceps brachii

f Pronator teres

g Teres major

h Brachialis

i Extensor carpi radialis

j Flexor carpi ulnaris

For each of the following questions, select the most appropriate answer from the above list of options. Each option may be used once, more than once or not at all.

1 Which nerve innervates elbow flexion?

2 Which nerve provides sensation to the medial one and a half digits?

3 Which nerve facilitates wrist extension?

4 Name a muscle that is supplied by the median nerve.

5 Name a muscle that is supplied by the ulnar nerve.

Theme: Anatomy of the lower limb

a   Sciatic nerve

b   Femoral nerve

c   Gastrocnemius

d   Tibialis anterior

e   Superior gluteal nerve

f   Inferior gluteal nerve

g   Obturator nerve

h   Tibial nerve

i   Deep peroneal nerve

j   Semitendinosus

For each of the following questions, select the most appropriate answer from the above list of options. Each option may be used once, more than once or not at all.

1   Which nerve innervates the hip flexors?

2   Name a muscle involved in hip extension.

3   Which nerve innervates the hip adductors?

4   Name a muscle involved in ankle dorsiflexion.

5   Which nerve innervates the gluteus maximus?

Section 3: Gastrointestinal and genitourinary systems

Single best answer

1 Which of the following arteries supply the midgut?

   a Superior mesenteric artery

   b Inferior mesenteric artery

   c Coeliac artery

   d Splenic artery

   e Left gastric artery

2 Which cells are responsible for the secretion of intrinsic factor?

   a Chief cells

   b Parietal cells

   c Islets of Langerhans

   d Acinar cells

   e Interstitial cells of Cajal

3   The following are all features of the large intestine EXCEPT:

   a   Splenic flexure

   b   Valvulae conniventes

   c   Haustra

   d   Vermiform appendix

   e   Caecum

4   Which of the following statements regarding the inguinal canal is correct?

   a   Its contents include the round ligament in women.

   b   The ilioinguinal nerve enters the canal via the deep ring.

   c   Abdominal contents herniating through the deep ring form a direct inguinal hernia.

   d   The inguinal canal is only present in males.

   e   The deep ring lies medial to the superficial inguinal ring.

5   Name the mesentery that anteriorly separates the right and left lobes of the liver.

   a   Quadrate mesentery

   b   Caudate mesentery

   c   Porta hepatis

   d   Hepatic mesentery

   e   Falciform ligament

6 Which three vessels branch from the coeliac trunk?

    a Common hepatic artery, superior mesenteric artery, inferior mesenteric artery

    b Left gastric artery, splenic artery, common hepatic artery

    c Cystic artery, splenic artery, gastric artery

    d Left gastric artery, common hepatic artery, superior mesenteric artery

    e Right hepatic artery, splenic artery, cystic artery

7 Which of the following vessels supply the distal third of the colon?

    a Left gastric artery

    b Common hepatic artery

    c Coeliac artery

    d Superior mesenteric artery

    e Inferior mesenteric artery

8 Which vessel originates in Calot's triangle?

    a Common hepatic artery

    b Hepatic vein

    c Cystic artery

    d Left gastric artery

    e Splenic artery

9 At which level does the superior mesenteric artery branch from the abdominal aorta?

a T11–T12

b L3–L4

c S1–S2

d L1–L2

e C8–T1

10 Which of the following most appropriately describes the position of the spleen?

a It is located in the right upper quadrant.

b It lies between the ninth and tenth ribs.

c It lies lateral to the right kidney.

d It is located between the third and fourth ribs.

e It lies between the tenth and twelfth ribs.

11 Which of the following statements is true with regard to the appendix?

a It is supplied by sympathetic and parasympathetic nerves from the superior mesenteric plexus.

b It lies behind the caecum in 5% of cases.

c It comprises taeniae coli similar to the caecum and colon.

d Options a, b and c are all incorrect.

e Options a, b and c are all correct.

12 Which of the following correctly identifies McBurney's point?

a Midway between the anterior superior iliac spine (ASIS) and the umbilicus

b Midway between the ASIS and the pubic symphysis

c At one-third of the distance from the right ASIS to the umbilicus

d At one-third of the distance from the right ASIS to the right pubic tubercle

e At two-thirds of the distance from the right ASIS to the umbilicus

13 The superior rectal artery is a branch of which vessel?

a Inferior mesenteric artery

b Coeliac artery

c Internal pudendal artery

d Internal iliac artery

e External iliac artery

14 The round ligament of the liver is an embryological remnant of which structure?

a Umbilical vein

b Umbilical artery

c Third branchial arch

d Falciform ligament

e Meckel's diverticulum

15 Which cells of the pancreas secrete somatostatin?

   a α-cells

   b β-cells

   c δ-cells

   d Acinar cells

   e Options a and b

16 The liver receives blood from which of the following?

   a Hepatic artery

   b Hepatic vein

   c Portal vein

   d Options a and c

   e Options a, b and c

17 Which of the following statements is correct with regard to the ampulla of Vater?

   a It is synonymous with the lower oesophageal sphincter.

   b It opens into the third part of the duodenum.

   c It is the point of entry of the accessory pancreatic duct into the duodenum.

   d It is the point of entry of the cystic duct into the second part of the duodenum.

   e It is the point of entry of the pancreatic duct and common bile duct into the duodenum.

18 The following statements are all correct with regard to the sigmoid colon EXCEPT:

a It is located in the right iliac fossa.

b It has a long mesentery.

c It is an intraperitoneal structure.

d It connects the descending colon to the rectum.

e It merges with the rectum at the level of S3.

19 The lower oesophageal sphincter is also known as which of the following?

a Cardiac sphincter

b Pyloric sphincter

c Sphincter of Oddi

d Glisson's sphincter

e Ileocaecal sphincter

20 The caecum overlies which of the following muscles?

a Sartorius

b Gluteus medius

c Iliacus

d Internal oblique

e None of the above

21 Which of the following is true with regard to Barrett's oesophagus?

   a A state where peristaltic movement of the oesophagus is inefficient.

   b There is dysfunction of the lower oesophageal sphincter.

   c There is achalasia of the oesophagus.

   d There is metaplasia: squamous to columnar epithelium.

   e There is metaplasia: columnar to squamous epithelium.

22 Which vessel supplies the tail of the pancreas?

   a Splenic artery

   b Superior pancreaticoduodenal artery

   c Inferior pancreaticoduodenal artery

   d Superior mesenteric artery

   e Inferior mesenteric artery

23 Which structure marks the division between autonomic and somatic innervation of the anal canal?

   a Anorectal junction

   b Venous anastomotic cushions

   c External sphincter

   d Dentate line

   e Internal sphincter

24 Which of the following statements is correct with regard to Meckel's diverticulum?

   a It is present in approximately 25% of the population.

   b It presents with left upper quadrant pain and haematemesis.

   c Perforation of Meckel's diverticulum may be mistaken for acute appendicitis.

   d It lies 2 cm proximal to the hepatic flexure of the transverse colon.

   e It is located in the distal colon and is a common cause of melaena.

25 Which of the following statements correctly differentiates the spleen from the kidney on examination?

   a The spleen has a characteristic 'notch'.

   b The spleen is ballotable, while the kidneys normally are not.

   c The kidneys descend on inspiration.

   d Options a, b and c are all incorrect.

   e Options a, b and c are all correct.

26 The vagina and uterus develop from which structure?

   a Mesonephric ducts

   b Ureteric bud

   c Wolffian ducts

   d Müllerian duct

   e Neural crest cells

27 The renal arteries divide into five vessels that enter each hilum. What is the name of these vessels?

   a Arcuate arteries

   b Interlobular arteries

   c Interlobar arteries

   d Segmental arteries

   e Lobar arteries

28 The blind end of the renal tubule and the site of filtration are known as which of the following?

   a Glomerulus

   b Bowman's capsule

   c Loop of Henle

   d Proximal tubule

   e Distal tubule

29 What type of epithelium lines the bladder?

   a Squamous

   b Pseudostratified columnar

   c Columnar

   d Stratified

   e Transitional

30 Which of the following best describes the position of the kidneys?

a C4–T1

b T2–T5

c T12–L3

d T4–T10

e L1–L4

31 Which vessel supplies the prostate?

a Inferior vesical artery

b Gonadal artery

c Internal iliac artery

d Testicular artery

e Right renal artery

32 Which muscle do the ureters overlie?

a Gracilis

b Sartorius

c Psoas

d Adductor magnus

e Quadriceps femoris

33 The fold of peritoneum formed between the uterus and rectum is known as which of the following?

a Pouch of Monro

b Uterosacral ligament

c Broad ligament

d Pouch of Douglas

e Enterocoele

34 The herniation of the bladder into the vagina (cystocele) can occur secondary to weakening of the pelvic floor muscles during childbirth. Which are the two main muscles of the pelvic floor?

a Transversus abdominis and rectus abdominis

b Obturator internus and internal oblique

c Levator ani and coccygeus

d Obturator internus and external oblique

e Coccygeus and transversus ani

35 Which of the following statements regarding the control of micturition is correct?

a The external urethral sphincter is a smooth muscle under sympathetic control.

b S2–S4 parasympathetic innervation results in contraction of the bladder.

c Sympathetic supply of the detrusor muscle stimulates micturition.

d The external urethral orifice lies posterior to the vaginal opening.

e Both internal and external sphincters are under voluntary control.

36 Vessels from which artery supply the penis?

a Inferior mesenteric artery

b Internal pudendal artery

c Internal iliac artery

d Internal inguinal artery

e External iliac artery

37 Under which of the following circumstances can the uterus be palpated abdominally at the level of the umbilicus?

   a During adulthood

   b Post menopause

   c When retroverted

   d Gravid uterus: at 12 weeks' gestation

   e Gravid uterus: at 20 weeks' gestation

38 The ridge in the peritoneum that nests the Fallopian tubes is known as which of the following?

   a Ovarian ligament

   b Round ligament

   c Broad ligament

   d Uterosacral ligament

   e Pouch of Douglas

39 To which vessel does the right gonadal vein drain?

   a Inferior vena cava

   b Right renal vein

   c Left renal vein

   d Right adrenal vein

   e Portal vein

40 Which is the narrowest part of the male urethra?

   a Intramural urethra

   b Proximal urethra

   c Spongy urethra

   d Membranous urethra

   e Prostatic urethra

Extended matching questions

Theme: Microanatomy of the gastrointestinal tract

a Parietal cells

b Chief cells

c Goblet cells

d Acinar cells

e Brunner's glands

f Pylorus

g Pepsin

h Hydrochloric acid

i Amylase

j α-cells

k β-cells

For each of the following questions, select the most appropriate answer from the above list of options. Each option may be used once, more than once or not at all.

1 Which pancreatic cells secrete glucagon?

2 Which cells secrete intrinsic factor, necessary for vitamin B_{12} absorption?

3 Name a substance secreted by the chief cells.

4 Name the exocrine cells of the pancreas.

5 Name the mucus-secreting cells of the duodenum.

Theme: Anatomy of the gastrointestinal tract

a   Ascending colon

b   Dorsal mesentery

c   Greater omentum

d   Lesser omentum

e   Haustra

f   Taeniae coli

g   Epiploic appendages

h   Diverticula

i   Descending colon

j   Transverse colon

k   Sigmoid colon

For each of the following questions, select the most appropriate answer from the above list of options. Each option may be used once, more than once or not at all.

1   Which intraperitoneal structure connects the right and left colic flexures?

2   Which structure connects the liver to the lesser curvature of the stomach?

3   Name the flat muscular bands of the large intestine.

4   Which part of the left side of the colon is intraperitoneal?

5   Name the pouches of viscera found on the large intestine.

Theme: Anatomy of the hepatobiliary system

   a Gall bladder

   b Liver

   c Pancreas

   d Erythrocytes

   e Bile duct

   f Hartmann's pouch

   g Cystic duct

   h Common bile duct

   i Hepatocytes

For each of the following questions, select the most appropriate answer from the above list of options. Each option may be used once, more than once or not at all.

1   The pancreatic duct joins with which other structure to enter the duodenum at the ampulla of Vater?

2   Which structure is found between the neck of the gall bladder and the cystic duct?

3   The hepatic duct joins with which structure to form the common bile duct?

4   Which structure is responsible for the formation of bile?

5   The breakdown of which structure results in the formation of unconjugated bilirubin?

Theme: Vasculature of the gastrointestinal system

a Median sacral artery

b Suprarenal artery

c Common iliac artery

d Lumbar arteries

e Left gastric artery

f Right gastric artery

g Coeliac artery

h Superior mesenteric artery

i Inferior mesenteric artery

For each of the following questions, select the most appropriate answer from the above list of options. Each option may be used once, more than once or not at all.

1 Which vessel has branches including left colic and sigmoid arteries?

2 Name a branch of the coeliac trunk.

3 Name the final unpaired branch of the abdominal aorta.

4 Name a vessel that branches off the abdominal aorta at the level of L1.

5 Name a vessel that originates at the level of L4.

Theme: Anatomy of hernias

a Richter's hernia

b Direct inguinal hernia

c Indirect inguinal hernia

d Femoral hernia

e Strangulated hernia

f Obstructed hernia

g Umbilical hernia

h Epigastric hernia

i Spigelian hernia

j Obturator hernia

For each of the following questions, select the most appropriate answer from the above list of options. Each option may be used once, more than once or not at all.

1 Which type of hernia occurs at the lateral edge of the rectus sheath?

2 Which type of hernia is found above and medial to the pubic tubercle and herniates through a defect in the abdominal wall fascia?

3 Which type of hernia is at risk of ischaemia due to an interruption in its blood supply?

4 Which type of hernia passes through the internal inguinal ring?

5 Which type of hernia is found lateral and inferior to the pubic tubercle?

Section 4: Cardiorespiratory system

Single best answer

1   Where is the bifurcation of the trachea (carina)?

   a   At the level of the atlanto-axial junction

   b   At the level of the C4–C5 intervertebral disc

   c   At the level of the T4–T5 intervertebral disc

   d   At the level of the cricothyroid cartilage

   e   Anterior to the lower oesophageal sphincter

2   Which valve separates the right atrium and right ventricle?

   a   Mitral

   b   Tricuspid

   c   Pulmonary

   d   Aortic

   e   Bicuspid

3 Which of the following correctly describes the position of the apex?

   a Second intercostal space, mid-axillary line

   b Fourth intercostal space, mid-axillary line

   c Fifth intercostal space, mid-axillary line

   d Third intercostal space, mid-clavicular line

   e Fifth intercostal space, mid-clavicular line

4 Which structure receives the four pulmonary veins?

   a Right atrium

   b Right ventricle

   c Left atrium

   d Left ventricle

   e Aortic arch

5 Name the main pacemaker region of the heart

   a Atrioventricular node

   b Purkinje fibres

   c Sinoatrial node

   d Interventricular septum

   e Bundle of His

6 Where is the oblique fissure found?

   a Left ventricle

   b Both lungs

   c Left lung

   d Right lung

   e Pulmonary trunk

7 Which of the following correctly defines the residual volume of the lung?

  a Total volume of the lungs after a maximal inspiratory effort

  b Volume of gas in the lungs after a maximal expiration

  c Amount of gas inhaled or exhaled during a normal breath

  d Volume of gas in the lungs after a normal expiration

  e Volume of gas that can be inhaled following a maximal inspiratory effort

8 Which of the following arteries supply the atrioventricular node in roughly 90% of people?

  a Ascending aorta

  b Posterior interventricular artery

  c Marginal artery

  d Left coronary artery

  e Left anterior descending artery

9 Which artery supplies the trachea?

  a Inferior thyroid artery

  b Cervical artery

  c Inferior laryngeal artery

  d Superior thyroid artery

  e Superior laryngeal artery

10 Which structure separates the left and right ventricles?

    a Aortic valve

    b Pulmonary valve

    c Tricuspid valve

    d Mitral valve

    e Interventricular septum

11 Which of the following statements concerning the great vessels is correct?

    a Branches of the aortic arch include the right common carotid, right subclavian and left brachiocephalic arteries.

    b Ligamentum arteriosum is an embryological remnant of the foramen ovale.

    c The right recurrent laryngeal nerve wraps around the ligamentum arteriosum, which is attached to the superior surface of the pulmonary trunk.

    d The common carotid arteries bifurcate into internal and external branches at the level of the superior border of the thyroid cartilage.

    e The external carotid artery lies posteriorly in the carotid sheath and its branches include the ophthalmic and inferior hypophyseal arteries.

12 At what level does the inferior vena cava pierce the diaphragm?

    a T6

    b Along with the thoracic duct through the oesophageal hiatus

    c T8

    d T10

    e Through the aortic hiatus at T12

13 A 50-year-old woman has recently returned from Ghana and presents to A&E with a 2-day history of rigors. A blood film demonstrates *Plasmodium falciparum* with a parasite count of 3%. On examination she is drowsy with a Glasgow Coma Scale score of 6/15, tachycardiac at 134 beats per minute and hypotensive at 60/55 mmHg. The medical registrar requests that a central line is inserted for aggressive fluid resuscitation. Which of the following statements regarding line insertion is NOT correct?

a The internal jugular vein is commonly used for central line placement and is used to monitor right atrial pressure.

b It can be used for parenteral feeding and the administration of drugs.

c The femoral vein is used preferentially because it has a lower risk of infection.

d The femoral vein lies medial to both the femoral artery and nerve.

e Complications of catheterising the subclavian vein include iatrogenic pneumothorax.

14 Which of the following statements regarding ventilation of the lungs is correct?

a The majority of ventilation occurs in the physiological dead space.

b The apices of the lungs are ventilated more efficiently than the bases.

c Some disease processes can reduce ventilation by decreasing dead space.

d A decrease in alveolar carbon dioxide is brought about by an increase in ventilation.

e The conducting airways are involved in gaseous exchange.

15 Which of the following vessels supply the airways?

    a Hilar pulmonary arteries

    b Bronchial arteries from the ascending aorta

    c Bronchial arteries from the descending thoracic aorta

    d Pulmonary artery

    e Pulmonary vein

16 Gases can move between adjacent alveoli through which structure?

    a Pores of Kohn

    b Type I pneumocytes

    c Type II pneumocytes

    d Mast cells

    e Erythrocytes

17 The space between the vocal cords changes shape in order to produce vocalisation. What is the correct name for this space?

    a Glottic compartment

    b Superior vestibular fold

    c Inferior vestibular fold

    d Supraglottis

    e Rima glottidis

18 Which substance is secreted by type II pneumocytes?

    a Mucus

    b Angiotensinogen

    c Renin

    d Angiotensin-converting enzyme

    e Surfactant

19 Which of the following statements regarding the anatomical development of the respiratory system is correct?

   a Surfactant develops from type I pneumocytes at week 28 to allow compliance of the alveoli.

   b The lungs begin to develop around the tenth week of gestation.

   c The mucosa of the respiratory system develops from an outpouching of the foregut endoderm.

   d Options a, b and c are all correct.

   e Options a, b and c are all incorrect.

20 Which of the following correctly identifies the position of the intercostal neurovascular bundle?

   a Midway between adjacent ribs

   b Directly above the rib

   c Directly below the rib

   d Between the fifth and sixth ribs

   e Along the subcostal margin

21 Which of the following statements regarding chest X-rays is correct?

   a The most prominent ribs on a chest X-ray are the posterior ribs.

   b The heart looks large on a posteroanterior film.

   c The left hemidiaphragm is higher than the right.

   d The left hilum is higher than the right.

   e The heart should be greater than half the width of the thorax for accurate interpretation.

22 Which of the following is NOT one of the four abnormalities of tetralogy of Fallot?

a Right ventricular hypertrophy

b Pulmonary stenosis

c Overriding aorta

d Dextrocardia

e Large ventricular septal defect

23 Which of the following is the most posterior structure of the heart?

a Left atrium

b Left ventricle

c Interventricular septum

d Right atrium

e Right ventricle

24 A stenotic aortic valve is likely to lead to which of the following?

a Right ventricular hypertrophy

b Left ventricular hypertrophy

c Right atrial hypertrophy

d Left ventricular dilation

e Left atrial hypertrophy

25 The P-wave of the electrocardiogram complex corresponds to which of the following?

a Mitral valve closure

b Atrial relaxation

c Atrial contraction

d Ventricular contraction

e Second heart sound

26 Which tumour most commonly occurs in the periphery of the lungs?

a Small cell carcinoma

b Squamous cell carcinoma

c Adenocarcinoma

d Alveolar cell carcinoma

e Large cell carcinoma

27 The following are all signs associated with Horner's syndrome EXCEPT:

a Chemosis

b Anhydrosis

c Miosis

d Mitosis

e Ptosis

28 Which of the following is a cause of Horner's syndrome?

   a Pancoast's tumour

   b Pneumothorax

   c Pleural effusion

   d Recurrent laryngeal nerve palsy

   e Tracheal tug

29 Tuberculosis infection results in chest X-ray changes in which part of the lung?

   a Hilar

   b Lung bases

   c Lung apices

   d Costophrenic angle

   e None of the above

30 The height of pulsation of which vessel is used to assess central venous pressure on cardiovascular examination?

   a External jugular vein

   b Internal jugular vein

   c Superior vena cava

   d Pulmonary vein

   e Pulmonary artery

31 Which vessel enters the right atrium of the heart?

   a Azygos vein

   b Pulmonary vein

   c Aorta

   d Pulmonary artery

   e Vena cava

32 Which of the following is a cause of bilateral hilar lymphadenopathy on a chest radiograph?

   a Unfolding aorta

   b Dextrocardia

   c Sarcoidosis

   d Situs inversus

   e Transposition of the great vessels

33 The following statements are all correct with regard to the pericardium EXCEPT:

   a The pericardium is located in the middle mediastinum.

   b The pericardium has fibrous and serous layers.

   c The pericardial sac encases the heart, which is surrounded by a small volume (approximately 50 mL) of fluid.

   d Pericardial sinuses exist between the pericardium and the surface of the heart.

   e The heart sits within the pericardium in the superior mediastinum.

34 Which of the following cranial bones make up part of the nasal septum?

   a Sphenoid

   b Ethmoid

   c Frontal

   d Options a and b

   e Options b and c

35 Which of the following nerves innervate the visceral pleura?

   a Intercostal nerves

   b Phrenic nerve

   c Anterior pulmonary plexus

   d Posterior pulmonary plexus

   e Options c and d

36 Which of the following statements regarding the anatomy of the foetal circulation is correct?

   a The umbilical vein transports deoxygenated blood from the foetus to the placenta.

   b At birth the umbilical vein fibrosis and its remnant is the ligamentum arteriosum, which attaches the umbilicus to the liver.

   c The falciform ligament of the liver separates left and right lobes and is the remnant of the umbilical vein.

   d The ductus venosus allows blood from the umbilical vein to bypass the foetal liver on its way to the inferior vena cava.

   e The ligamentum teres is located on the underside of the liver and is the embryological remnant of the umbilical artery.

37 A branchial cyst is an embryological remnant of a branchial cleft, which presents as a cystic mass in the anterior triangle of the neck. Which of the following statements regarding the anatomy of the neck is NOT correct?

a The anterior triangle contains the submandibular lymph nodes and hypoglossal nerve.

b The sternal head of the sternocleidomastoid muscle attaches to the manubrium, while its clavicular head is attached to the medial third of the clavicle.

c The maxillary and superficial temporal arteries are the terminal branches of the external carotid artery.

d Platysma is supplied by the cervical branch of the facial nerve (cranial nerve VII).

e The medial border of the sternocleidomastoid muscle, the clavicle and the trapezius muscle form the borders of the anterior triangle.

38 Surfactant is a detergent-like complex that lines the alveoli and is responsible for lung compliance. Neonates born prematurely lack surfactant and consequently can develop respiratory distress syndrome. Which of the following cells are responsible for surfactant production?

a Type I pneumocytes

b Type II pneumocytes

c Alveolar macrophages

d B-lymphocytes

e T-lymphocytes

39 A 78-year-old lifelong smoker presents with pain in his right shoulder, weight loss and haemoptysis. On further questioning he admits to weakness of the muscles in his right hand and on examination exhibits evidence of Horner's syndrome. What is the most likely diagnosis?

   a Lower lobe pneumonia

   b Lower lobe cancer

   c Laryngopharyngeal carcinoma

   d Pneumothorax

   e Apical (Pancoast's) tumour

40 Which one of the following statements concerning the coronary vessels is correct?

   a Maximal flow through the coronary arteries occurs during systole.

   b A proportion of blood through the coronary vessels shunts directly to the right side of the heart.

   c Parasympathetic innervation causes dilation of the coronary vessels.

   d The atrioventricular node is supplied by the left coronary artery in around 90% of people.

   e The coronary vessels drain into the coronary sinus, which runs in the anterior interventricular groove.

Extended matching questions

Theme: Cardiac structure and function

- a Mitral stenosis
- b Pulmonary valve
- c Mitral regurgitation
- d Tricuspid valve
- e Aortic valve
- f Bicuspid valve
- g Semilunar valve
- h Chordae tendineae

For each of the following questions, select the most appropriate answer from the above list of options. Each option may be used once, more than once or not at all.

1 The mitral valve is an example of which type of valve?

2 Which valvular abnormality can be heard as a pansystolic murmur loudest at the apex?

3 Which structure separates the right atrium and ventricle?

4 Which of the above options is most commonly associated with atrial fibrillation?

5 Which valve prevents blood flowing back into the left ventricle?

Theme: Anatomy of the great vessels

a   Pulmonary vein

b   Vena cava

c   Aortic arch

d   Subclavian artery

e   Brachiocephalic artery

f   Common carotid artery

g   Vertebral artery

h   Pulmonary artery

For each of the following questions, select the most appropriate answer from the above list of options. Each option may be used once, more than once or not at all.

1   Which vessel carries oxygenated blood from the lungs to the left atrium?

2   Which vessel branches from the aortic arch to form the common carotid and subclavian artery?

3   Which vessel carries blood away from the right ventricle?

4   Which vessel divides at the superior border of the thyroid to form internal and external branches?

5   Which structure provides the following three branches: left subclavian, left common carotid and brachiocephalic arteries?

Theme: Anatomy of the larynx

a Arytenoid cartilage

b Thyrohyoid

c Epiglottis

d Hyoid

e Cricothyroid

f Thyroid cartilage

g Cricoid cartilage

h Thymus

i Thyroarytenoid

For each of the following questions, select the most appropriate answer from the above list of options. Each option may be used once, more than once or not at all.

1 Name a structure of the superior mediastinum.

2 Which muscle tightens the vocal cords and is supplied by the superior laryngeal nerve?

3 Which U-shaped bone is at the level of C3–C4?

4 Which muscle connects the hyoid bone to the larynx?

5 Name the structure inferior to the thyroid cartilage and shaped like a signet ring.

Theme: Relations of the diaphragm

   a Vagus nerve

   b Phrenic nerve

   c Intercostal nerve

   d C8

   e T2

   f T4

   g T6

   h T8

   i T10

   j T12

For each of the following questions, select the most appropriate answer from the above list of options. Each option may be used once, more than once or not at all.

1   At which level does the oesophagus pierce the diaphragm?

2   At which level does the angle of Louis lie?

3   Which nerve supplies the diaphragm?

4   At which level does the aorta pierce the diaphragm?

5   At which level does the vena cava pierce the diaphragm?

Theme: Anatomy of the airways

a Epiglottis

b Cilia

c Lingular lobe

d Carina

e Terminal bronchiole

f Trachea

g Alveoli

h Bronchial artery

i Middle lobe

For each of the following questions, select the most appropriate answer from the above list of options. Each option may be used once, more than once or not at all.

1 Which vessel supplies the distal airways?

2 Which structure is located between the left upper and lower lobes of the lung?

3 What is the name of the most distal part of the airways?

4 The bifurcation of the trachea is known by which other name?

5 Which structure protects the airway on swallowing?

Answers

Section 1: Neuroanatomy

1 d

The spinothalamic tract is an ascending spinal tract that carries the modalities of temperature and pain as well as pressure and non-discriminative touch. Spinal cord lesions result in loss of pain and temperature sensation on the contralateral side of the body. This is because the spinothalamic tract crosses close to its origin via the ventral white commissure. The dorsal columns carry information related to vibration sense, discriminative touch and proprioception. As the primary afferent neurons ascend to the medulla oblongata before decussation, spinal cord lesions result in ipsilateral loss of the dorsal column modalities.

2 e

The olfactory nerve passes through the cribriform plate of the ethmoid bone to the olfactory bulb on the inferior aspect of the frontal lobe. The fibres pass along the olfactory tract to the primary olfactory cortex of the uncus. Anosmia is the inability to smell and can occur secondary to head trauma or space-occupying lesions, e.g. meningioma.

3 a

The glossopharyngeal nerve (cranial nerve IX) innervates taste to the posterior third of the tongue, while the facial nerve (cranial nerve VII) supplies taste to the anterior two-thirds. The glossopharyngeal nerve conveys sensation from the pharynx to mediate the gag reflex and its small motor component innervates the stylopharyngeus muscle, which facilitates swallowing.

4 a

The termination of the spinal cord occurs at the level of the L1–L2 disc in adult life. For this reason, procedures such as lumbar punctures and epidural injections can be safely performed caudal to the L1–L2 disc.

5 a

The brain is covered by three membranous layers called the meninges: dura, arachnoid and pia mater. The space outside of the dura, the extradural layer, contains the middle meningeal artery. Trauma can lead to tearing of the artery, causing blood to accumulate in the extradural space. Burr hole surgery is required to prevent fatal compression of the brain. An extradural haematoma is diagnosed by a convex shape on a computerised tomography scan, while a subdural bleed is crescentic or concave in shape.

6 a

The facial nerve supplies the muscles of facial expression, which include the stylohyoid, platysma and digastric muscles, as well as the stapedius in the middle ear. The facial nerve causes contraction of the stapedius in response to loud sounds and prior to speech, acting as a protective mechanism. This attenuates the movement of the stapes in the oval window and thus reduces cochlea auditory input.

7 c

The posterior cerebral artery branches from the basilar artery to supply the occipital lobe. The anterior and middle cerebral arteries branch from the internal carotid artery at the level of the optic chiasm. The anterior cerebral arteries supply the medial aspect of the hemispheres, while the middle cerebral arteries supply the lateral aspect.

8 b

The posterior pituitary, or neurohypophysis, is responsible for the secretion of oxytocin and antidiuretic hormone. Oxytocin is involved in birth and lactation, while antidiuretic hormone is responsible for the control of plasma osmolarity. It is secreted in response to high plasma osmolarity, in order to conserve water at the collecting duct of the nephron.

9 c

The corneal reflex can be elicited by tactile stimulation of the cornea, via the ophthalmic branch of the trigeminal nerve, or by bright light, via the optic nerve. The efferent limb is supplied by the facial nerve, which causes a brief contraction of the orbicularis oculi, protecting the cornea and retina from trauma and exposure to bright light.

10 a

Corticobulbar fibres innervating the muscles of the upper face, e.g. orbicularis oculi and frontalis, are distributed bilaterally. A unilateral lesion to these fibres (i.e. upper motor neuron lesion) causes weakness of the lower facial muscles only. A lower motor neuron lesion of the facial nerve causes complete unilateral weakness of the face. Asking the patient to raise their eyebrows allows for differentiation between the two types.

11 a

The trigeminal nerve comprises three branches: ophthalmic, maxillary and mandibular. It conveys sensation of pain, temperature, pressure and touch of the face, in addition to supplying the muscles of mastication. The entry and exit foramina of the cranial nerves represent potential sites of trauma and compression. Each of the three branches traverses different foramina. The first is the ophthalmic branch, which passes through the superior orbital fissure; the second is the maxillary branch, which traverses the foramen rotundum; the third is the mandibular branch, which passes through the foramen ovale.

12 a

The extraocular muscles, excluding the superior oblique and the lateral rectus, are innervated by the oculomotor nerve. Action of the lateral rectus is responsible for lateral gaze and is supplied by the abducens nerve, while the superior oblique facilitates infero-medial movement of the eye and is supplied by the trochlear nerve.

13 b

The internal carotid artery divides into its two terminal branches at the level of the optic chiasm: the anterior cerebral and middle cerebral arteries. The anterior cerebral artery supplies the anterior and medial brain. The anterior communicating artery connects the two anterior cerebral arteries to form the anterior portion of the circle of Willis.

14 b

Tearing of the veins in the subdural space can cause accumulation of blood. Since the blood collects slowly, there may be a delay between the mechanism of injury and the onset of symptoms. Older people at risk of falls commonly present late with subdural haematomas, which can lead to coma and death.

15 c

The basal ganglia are involved in the control of movement and posture. The main components are the striatum (caudate nucleus and putamen) and the globus pallidus. The mammillary bodies project to the anterior thalamic nuclei as part of the limbic system.

16 d

Compression of the optic chiasm can occur secondary to a pituitary tumour and results in a bitemporal hemianopia. At the chiasm, fibres from the nasal half of the retina decussate before entering the optic tracts, thus information from the temporal fields is lost and results in a bitemporal hemianopia.

17 b

The superior oblique is innervated by the trochlear nerve and facilitates infero-medial movement of the eye. The lateral rectus facilitates lateral movement of the eye and is supplied by the abducens nerve. The remainder of the extraocular muscles are supplied by the oculomotor nerve.

18 d

The cranial nerves supply ipsilateral structures. The hypoglossal nerve (cranial nerve XII) provides motor supply to the intrinsic muscles of the tongue. A lower motor neuron lesion to this nerve results in wasting on the ipsilateral side and deviation of the tongue towards the side of the lesion.

19 c

The foramina of the middle cranial fossa run infero-laterally and can be remembered by the mnemonic '**R**eview **O**f **S**ystems':

- foramen **R**otundum – maxillary branch of trigeminal
- foramen **O**vale – mandibular branch of trigeminal
- foramen **S**pinosum – middle meningeal artery.

20 b

The motor branches of the trigeminal nerve supply the muscles of mastication. See table for an outline of the three basic sensory divisions and corresponding foramina.

Nerve	Sensation	Cranial foramina
Ophthalmic branch	Scalp, forehead, nose, cornea and conjunctivae	Superior orbital fissure
Maxillary branch	Lower eyelid, cheek, upper lip, upper teeth and gums	Foramen rotundum
Mandibular branch	Lower lip, lower teeth, chin and jaw	Foramen ovale

21 a

The common carotid divides into internal and external branches at the level of the superior border of the thyroid. The ophthalmic artery branches at the level of the anterior clinoid process, which enters the orbit via the optic canal. The two terminal branches of the internal carotid join the vertebrobasilar system to form the circle of Willis.

22 a

The dorsal columns are the ascending spinal tracts that carry information related to the sensory modalities of proprioception and fine touch. The first-order neurons ascend ipsilaterally to the medulla, terminating at the nucleus gracilis and nucleus cuneatus. Second-order neurons decussate as the internal arcuate fibres and then ascend to the thalamus as the medial lemniscus. The tract is completed by third-order neurons that travel to the somatosensory cortex.

23 b

Cerebrospinal fluid (CSF) is produced by the choroid plexus of the ventricular system. Approximately 150 mL of CSF bathes the brain and the spinal cord. CSF leaves the fourth ventricle through the foramina of Magendie and Luschka to enter the subarachnoid space.

24 d

The postcentral gyrus is part of the parietal lobe and is located immediately posterior to the central sulcus. The postcentral gyrus hosts the primary somatosensory cortex, while the precentral gyrus is functionally known as the primary motor cortex.

25 d

The three principle neuroglial cells are oligodendrocytes, astrocytes and microglia. Oligodendrocytes are responsible for the production of myelin. Astrocytes play a role in the formation of the blood–brain barrier, while the microglia act as phagocytes of the nervous system.

26 c

In an UPPER motor neuron lesion, both tone and reflexes INCREASE and plantar responses are UP-going.

Upper motor neuron lesion	Lower motor neuron lesion
Weakness	Weakness
Wasting (chronic)	Wasting (acute)
Increased tone	Decreased tone
Increased reflexes	Decreased reflexes
Up-going plantar responses	Down-going plantar responses

27 c

The two hormones secreted from the posterior pituitary are oxytocin and antidiuretic hormone (ADH). ADH acts on the collecting duct of the nephron to conserve water by increasing its permeability and therefore water reabsorption. A reduction in the secretion or action of ADH results in diabetes insipidus, in which the nephron is unable to concentrate the urine in order to conserve body water. This results in symptoms of profound thirst and polyuria.

28 c

Directly anterior to the central sulcus in the frontal lobe is the precentral gyrus, the primary motor cortex. The primary motor cortex controls voluntary motor control of the contralateral side of the body.

29 d

Vitamin B_{12} deficiency can result from absorption disorders such as short bowel syndrome and pernicious anaemia. Pernicious anaemia occurs in the presence of anti-parietal cell or anti-intrinsic factor antibodies, and is associated with impaired vitamin B_{12} absorption. In addition to weakness and spasticity, subacute combined degeneration of the cord results in sensory ataxia.

30 d

Visual field defects are commonly tested in exams:
- optic nerve lesion – ipsilateral monocular blindness
- optic chiasm lesion – bitemporal hemianopia

- Temporal lobe lesion – contralateral **S**uperior quadrantanopia (remember '**ST**')
- parietal lobe lesion – contralateral inferior quadrantanopia
- anterior circulation stroke – homonymous hemianopia.

31 d

The mnemonic '**T**o **Z**anzibar **B**y **M**otor **C**ar' can be used to remember the five major branches of the facial nerve:
- **T**emporal branch
- **Z**ygomatic branch
- **B**uccal branch
- **M**arginal mandibular branch
- **C**ervical branch.

32 b

Broca's area is located in the frontal lobe in the inferior frontal gyrus. It controls the expression of language and speech. Wernicke's area, the auditory association cortex, is situated in the temporal lobe and is responsible for comprehension of language.

33 e

Charcot's triad is made up of dysarthria, nystagmus and intention tremor and is indicative of a cerebellar lesion. The acronym 'DANISH' can be used to remember the signs of cerebellar disease:
- **D**ysdiadochokinesia
- **A**taxia
- **N**ystagmus
- **I**ntention tremor
- **S**lurred speech
- **H**ypotonia.

34 b

Parkinson's disease is thought to occur secondary to loss of dopaminergic transmission in the nigrostriatal pathway, in the presence of Lewy bodies. L-dopa, the dopamine precursor, is used along with a decarboxylase inhibitor, which prevents the peripheral breakdown of l-dopa, in the control of symptoms.

35 e

The spinal branch of the accessory nerve supplies the sternoclei-domastoid and trapezius muscles. These muscles facilitate lateral rotation of the neck and shoulder elevation, respectively.

36 e

Cerebrospinal fluid (CSF) is formed in the choroid plexus, mostly in the lateral ventricle. From here, CSF passes through the foramen of Monro to the third ventricle. The cerebral aqueduct connects the third and fourth ventricles, from which CSF enters the subarachnoid space and passes through the central canal to line the spinal cord.

37 c

Wernicke's encephalopathy occurs secondary to thiamine deficiency, e.g. in alcohol-dependent patients. Urgent thiamine replacement is needed to prevent the progression to Korsakoff's syndrome, an irreversible condition resulting in amnesia and confabulation.

38 d

The internal carotid artery enters the cranium via the foramen lacerum. Its terminal two branches, the anterior and middle cerebral arteries, join the posterior cerebral artery from the vertebrobasilar system to form the circle of Willis.

39 d

The foramen magnum is the largest foramen of the posterior cranial fossa. The medulla passes through the foramen magnum continuous with the spinal cord. The vertebral arteries and spinal part of the accessory nerve also pass through the foramen magnum. The hypoglossal canal lies in the lateral wall of the foramen, through which the hypoglossal nerve travels.

40 a

The primary visual cortex is located in the gyri directly above and below the calcarine sulcus on the medial side of the occipital lobe.

Theme: Where is the lesion?

1 c

2 a

3 j

4 h

5 b

Visual defects are easy points in exams if you understand the anatomy behind the pathology. A stroke affecting the temporal lobe results in a superior quadrantanopia, while a parietal lobe infarct results in an inferior quadrantanopia. Because the fibres carrying information from the lateral field decussate at the optic chiasm, a chiasm lesion (e.g. pituitary tumour) results in tunnel vision or bitemporal hemianopia. All the extraocular muscles are supplied by the oculomotor nerve (cranial nerve III), except for two: the superior oblique, supplied by the trochlear (IV) nerve, and the lateral rectus, supplied by the abducens (VI) nerve. The pupillary light reflex involves both the optic (II) and oculomotor (III) nerves. Stimulation of the optic nerve results in consensual pupillary constriction via both oculomotor nerves. Shining a light into the right eye causes activation of the right optic nerve. With all nerves intact, both pupils should constrict via efferent signals from both oculomotor nerves.

Theme: Anatomy of the cranial foramina

1 f

2 b

3 h

4 d

5 a

Compression or a lesion anywhere along the course of the nerve can result in subsequent deficit. A common place for injury is where the nerve passes through its cranial foramina.

Nerve	Cranial foramina
Olfactory	Cribriform plate
Optic	Optic canal
Oculomotor	Superior orbital fissure
Trochlear	Superior orbital fissure
Trigeminal	I: superior orbital fissure II: foramen rotundum III: foramen ovale
Abducens	Superior orbital fissure
Facial	Stylohyoid foramen
Vestibulocochlear	Internal auditory meatus
Glossopharyngeal	Jugular foramen
Vagus	Jugular foramen
Accessory	Cranial: jugular foramen Spinal: foramen magnum
Hypoglossal	Hypoglossal canal

Theme: Neuroendocrinology

1 d

2 h

3 c

4 f

5 c

The anterior pituitary is responsible for the secretion of all but two pituitary hormones.

Hormones of the anterior pituitary	Hormones of the posterior pituitary
Follicle-stimulating hormone	Oxytocin
Luteinising hormone	Antidiuretic hormone
Adrenocorticotrophic hormone	
Prolactin	
Thyroid-stimulating hormone	

Theme: Anatomy of the spinal tracts

1 f

2 d

3 b

4 c

5 h

The spinal tracts are divided into ascending and descending. Ascending tracts carry sensory information from peripheral receptors to the cortex. The dorsal columns carry proprioception, vibration and discriminative touch to the somatosensory cortex. The tracts cross in the medulla as the internal arcuate fibres. The spinothalamic tract is another ascending tract, which carries the modalities of temperature and pain. Fibres of the spinothalamic tracts cross to the contralateral side of the cord within one or two spinal segments. The descending tracts carry fibres from the cortex and are involved with the control of movement and posture. Examples include the corticospinal, rubrospinal and vestibulospinal tracts.

Theme: Anatomy of the cranial nerves

1 a

2 b

3 f

4 d

5 a

The trigeminal nerve (cranial nerve V) is divided into three branches, providing sensation to the face and motor function to the muscles of mastication. They include the temporalis, masseter and lateral and medial pterygoids. The glossopharyngeal nerve (cranial nerve IX) provides taste to the posterior one-third of the tongue; the facial nerve (cranial nerve VII) provides taste to the anterior two-thirds. The afferent limb of the pupillary light reflex is the optic nerve (cranial nerve II). Stimulation results in consensual constriction of both pupils via the efferent limb, the oculomotor nerve (cranial nerve III). The spinal component of the accessory nerve (cranial nerve XI) innervates the sternocleidomastoid and trapezius muscles. Finally, the afferent limb of the corneal reflex is provided by the ophthalmic branch of the trigeminal nerve upon tactile stimulation of the cornea. This reflex can also be initiated via the optic nerve in response to bright light.

Section 2: Musculoskeletal system

1 d

Dislocation of the gleno-humeral joint usually occurs anteriorly (typically 95% of cases). The course of the axillary nerve makes it particularly vulnerable. Classically, axillary nerve lesions result in loss of an area of sensation on the upper arm that corresponds to the position of the regimental badge on a military uniform. As the axillary nerve supplies the deltoid and teres minor, injury also results in weakness of shoulder abduction.

2 c

The deep inguinal ring lies midway between the pubic **tubercle** and anterior superior iliac spine – that is, midway along the inguinal ligament. This is often confused with the mid-inguinal point, which corresponds to the position of the femoral artery. The mid-inguinal point is located halfway between the anterior superior iliac spine and the pubic **symphysis**.

3 b

The long thoracic nerve innervates the serratus anterior muscle. Damage to this nerve classically results in 'winging' of the scapula.

4 b

The rotator cuff both protects and facilitates movement at the shoulder joint. The acronym 'SITS' can be used to remember the four muscles that make up the rotator cuff:
- **S**upraspinatus
- **I**nfraspinatus
- **T**eres minor
- **S**ubscapularis.

5 c

The posterior tibial artery branches from the popliteal artery and runs to the flexor compartment of the lower leg. It can be palpated behind the medial malleolus.

6 a

Flexor digitorum profundus attaches distally to the flexor digitorum superficialis, which facilitates movement at the proximal interphalangeal joint. The flexor digitorum profundus contracts to flex the distal interphalangeal joint.

7 a

The ulnar nerve supplies all the small muscles of the hand except for 'LOAF', which are supplied by the median nerve:
- **L**ateral two lumbricals
- **O**pponens pollicis
- **A**bductor pollicis brevis
- **F**lexor pollicis brevis.

The median nerve also supplies the quadratus and pronator teres.

8 d

The femoral triangle contains the femoral nerve, artery and vein. It is bordered by the adductor longus muscle, inguinal ligament and sartorius muscle.

9 a

The acronym 'NAVY' can be used to remember the structures, located from lateral to medial, inside the femoral triangle:

- femoral **N**erve
- femoral **A**rtery
- femoral **V**ein
- deep inguinal l**Y**mph nodes.

10 a

Sensation of the hand is provided by the median, ulnar and radial nerves. The ulnar nerve supplies the medial one and a half digits and the median nerve supplies the remainder. The radial nerve supplies a small area on the dorsum of the hand over the first interphalangeal web space.

11 d

The hamstrings are made up of three muscles: semimembranosus, semitendinosus and biceps femoris. They facilitate hip flexion and knee extension and are supplied by the sciatic nerve.

12 c

Carpal tunnel syndrome results in compression of the median nerve between the carpal bones and flexor retinaculum. Causes of carpal tunnel syndrome include acromegaly, rheumatoid arthritis and hypothyroidism.

13 e

The common iliac artery bifurcates into internal and external branches at the level of the sacroiliac joints. The external iliacs supply the lower limbs, while the internal iliac arteries supply the pelvis and reproductive organs.

14 d

The brachial pulse can be palpated medial to the biceps tendon in the antecubital fossa. The brachial artery divides into the radial and ulnar arteries to supply the forearm.

15 b

The gleno-humeral joint is stabilised by the rotator cuff muscles: teres minor, subscapularis, supraspinatus and infraspinatus. Dislocation usually occurs antero-inferiorly and can result in damage to the axillary nerve.

16 c

The popliteal artery is derived from the femoral artery and divides into two branches: anterior and posterior tibial arteries. The anterior tibial descends along the interosseous membrane to supply the anterior lower leg and then becomes the dorsalis pedis artery, which supplies the forefoot.

17 a

The extensor digitorum longus, extensor hallucis and tibialis anterior all facilitate ankle dorsiflexion. The gastrocnemius, soleus, tibialis posterior and flexor digitorum longus are all plantar flexors.

18 c

A sesamoid bone is a bone that lies within a tendon. Examples include the patella, which lies within the quadriceps tendon, and the pisiform metacarpal, located in the flexor carpi ulnaris muscle.

19 e

The knee joint is a hinge synovial joint, protected by a capsule and strengthened by ligaments. These include the medial and lateral collateral ligaments and anterior and posterior cruciate ligaments.

20 e

The thoracodorsal nerve supplies the latissimus dorsi muscle, which facilitates shoulder extension and adduction. The latissimus dorsi (meaning 'broadest muscle of the back') attaches to the spinous processes of T7–T12. It inserts into the intertubercular groove of the humerus between the pectoralis major and teres major muscles.

21 a

The ligaments of the spinal column can be divided into short and long ligaments. The long ligaments include anterior longitudinal, posterior longitudinal and supraspinous ligaments, while the short ligaments are ligamentum flava, intertransverse and interspinous ligaments. Ligamentum flava joins adjacent lamina, the intertransverse ligaments extend between transverse processes and interspinous ligaments join adjacent spinous processes.

22 a

The sartorius (from the Latin *sartor*, meaning 'tailor') muscle facilitates sitting cross-legged – classically the position in which tailors sat to work. It is supplied by the femoral nerve and forms the lateral border of the femoral triangle.

23 d

The quadriceps muscles facilitate knee extension and are made up of the rectus femoris, vastus medialis, vastus intermedius and vastus lateralis. The semitendinosus, on the other hand, is one of the hamstring muscles and is supplied by the sciatic nerve.

24 c

The femoral nerve supplies the quadriceps muscles. It also sends branches to the iliacus, pectineus and sartorius muscles.

25 e

The common carotid artery divides into internal and external branches at the superior border of the thyroid cartilage. The internal carotid artery ascends in the carotid sheath. It forms the tortuous carotid syphon and passes through the foramen lacerum. Along its course the internal carotid supplies the middle ear and posterior pituitary, and also branches to form the ophthalmic artery and the central artery of the retina. Its two terminal branches are the anterior and middle cerebral arteries, which join with the vertebrobasilar system to form the circle of Willis.

26 c

The masseter, pterygoids and temporalis are the muscles of mastication supplied by the trigeminal nerve (cranial nerve V). The lateral pterygoid aids in depressing the mandible and thereby facilitates opening the jaw.

27 a

The dorsalis pedis artery stems from the anterior tibial artery. It runs over the dorsum of the foot and is usually palpable in the second web space. It supplies the toes through its dorsal metacarpal and arcuate branches.

28 c

The course of the round ligament of the uterus, or ligamentum teres, follows that of the spermatic cord in men, passing through the deep ring, along the inguinal canal and into the labia majora.

29 b

The patella tendon is the termination of the quadriceps and attaches to the patella itself. The patella ligament, on the other hand, attaches to the tibial tuberosity.

30 d

C5 innervates the biceps jerk reflex, C6 innervates the brachioradialis and C7 innervates the triceps reflex. Stretching the tendon activates stretch receptors and initiates the reflex arc. Efferents in the anterior horn signal to the muscle and result in contraction.

31 c

Dislocation of the femoral head usually occurs posteriorly, which puts the sciatic nerve at risk of injury. Sciatic nerve lesions can produce pain in the buttocks that is referred down the leg. Damage to the sciatic nerve is a cause of foot-drop.

32 b

The anatomy of the brachial plexus is important clinically and it often comes up in exams. The lateral cord forms the musculocutaneous nerve, and joins with the medial cord to form the median nerve.

33 b

Upon nociceptive stimulation of the lateral border of the foot, a normal individual will have a plantar flexion response. In an upper motor neuron lesion – that is, damage to the spinal cord or to the cortex itself – there is an 'up-going' response (a positive Babinski reflex).

34 a

The first vertebra (C1) is known as the atlas vertebra, named after the Titan in Greek mythology who was forced to support the heavens on his shoulders. It is made up of anterior and posterior arches, with a lateral mass, containing the foramen transversarium, through which the vertebral artery passes.

35 d

A Baker's cyst is a benign swelling of the semimembranous bursa in the popliteal fossa. A ruptured Baker's cyst results in calf pain and swelling. However, a deep-vein thrombosis is an important differential diagnosis.

36 b

The recurrent laryngeal nerve supplies all of the intrinsic muscles of the larynx apart from the cricothyroid. The cricothyroid muscle lies on the external aspect of the larynx, attaching from the lateral aspect of the cricoid arch to the thyroid lamina. Unlike the other laryngeal muscles, it is supplied by the external laryngeal branch of the superior laryngeal nerve.

37 e

The scaphoid carpal bone is prone to fracture upon falling on an out-stretched hand. Because it is supplied from its distal end, interruption of its blood supply secondary to improper healing can lead to avascular necrosis of its proximal segment.

38 b

The radial artery passes through the 'anatomical snuffbox' to supply the superficial and deep palmar arches. The 'anatomical snuffbox' has boundaries comprising the extensor pollicis longus, extensor pollicis brevis and abductor pollicis longus muscles.

39 b

C2, known as the 'axis vertebra', can be recognised by the presence of the odontoid peg. The odontoid peg articulates with the anterior arch of C1, the 'atlas vertebra'. Fractures of the odontoid peg can result in damage to the cervical cord.

40 d

The knee joint is a hinge synovial joint surrounded by a protective capsule. The collateral and cruciate ligaments strengthen the joint. The prepatellar and suprapatellar bursae facilitate movement and protect the joint.

Theme: Anatomy of the hand

1 g

2 k

3 e

4 j

5 k

The anatomy of the hand is very intricate. For preclinical and final examinations, the basics are most likely to be tested. The sensory divisions of the hand are commonly examined: the medial three and a half digits are supplied by the median nerve and the lateral one and a half are supplied by the ulnar. To test the radial nerve, sensation over the first web space on the dorsum of the hand can be examined.

Theme: Blood supply of the upper limbs

1 g

2 f

3 l

4 e

5 i

The upper limbs are supplied bilaterally by the subclavian arteries. The left subclavian artery branches directly off the aortic arch; the right subclavian artery, along with the right common carotid artery, branches from the brachiocephalic artery. On passing under the clavicle the subclavian becomes the axillary artery, which in turn becomes the brachial artery. The brachial artery can be palpated in the antecubital fossa.

Theme: Blood supply of the lower limbs

1 a

2 j

3 f

4 g

5 d

The external iliac arteries and their subsequent branches supply the legs. Venous drainage occurs via the long and short saphenous veins. The long saphenous vein runs along the medial aspect of the limb and drains into the femoral vein at the saphenous opening of the fascia lata. The superficial and deep systems are connected by the communicating veins.

Theme: Anatomy of the upper limb

1 c

2 b

3 c

4 f

5 j

The biceps, brachialis and brachioradialis facilitate elbow flexion, while the triceps facilitate elbow extension. The median nerve supplies the pronator teres and quadratus, which facilitates pronation, while the radial nerve innervates the supinator and brachioradialis.

Theme: Anatomy of the lower limb

1 b

2 j

3 g

4 d

5 a

Flexion of the hip is brought about by the quadriceps, supplied by the femoral nerve. The quadriceps (rectus femoris, vastus medialis, vastus intermedius and vastus lateralis) also facilitate knee extension. Hip extensors and knee flexors are mainly supplied by the sciatic nerve and comprise the hamstring muscles: semimembranosus, semitendinosus and biceps femoris.

Section 3: Gastrointestinal and genitourinary systems

1 a

During development the alimentary canal is divided into the foregut, midgut and hindgut. It is supplied by three major unpaired vessels that arise from the abdominal aorta. The coeliac trunk supplies the foregut – that is, the gut proximal to the major duodenal papilla. At this point the midgut commences, ending about two-thirds of the way along the transverse colon, and is supplied by the superior mesenteric artery. The distal gut is supplied by the inferior mesenteric artery.

2 b

Parietal cells of the stomach are responsible for the secretion of intrinsic factor, which is necessary for the absorption of vitamin B_{12}. Pernicious anaemia occurs in the presence of auto-antibodies against intrinsic factor and/or parietal cells themselves. Macrocytic anaemia occurs secondary to vitamin B_{12} deficiency.

3 b

The large intestine is made up of four sections: the appendix and caecum, colon, rectum and anal canal. The colon is separated into ascending, transverse, descending and sigmoid, from proximal to distal. Distinguishing features of the large intestine include the taeniae coli, epiploic appendices and haustra.

4 a

The inguinal canal runs infero-medially between the deep and superficial inguinal rings. It develops embryologically to allow for descent of the testes into the scrotal sac, by the shortening of the gubernaculum, which attaches the gonads to the labioscrotal swellings. In the absence of male hormones, the gubernaculum persists and its remnant is known as the round ligament. In addition to the spermatic cord or round ligament, the inguinal canal also contains the ilioinguinal nerve. Because the ilioinguinal nerve enters via the superficial ring, it passes through only part of the canal and supplies sensation to the root of the penis and upper scrotum or mons pubis and labia majora. An indirect hernia forms when abdominal contents protrude through the deep ring, whereas a **direct hernia** bypasses the canal and herniates **directly** through the abdominal wall fascia.

5 e

The liver is divided into four lobes: right, left, caudate and quadrate. The falciform ligament divides the right and left lobes. The umbilical fissure contains the ligamentum teres, the embryological remnant of the umbilical vein.

6 b

The coeliac trunk is the first unpaired branch of the abdominal aorta. It supplies the foregut, and its three branches are the left gastric, splenic and common hepatic arteries.

7 e

The inferior mesenteric artery supplies the hindgut derivatives – that is, from the distal third of the transverse colon to the anal canal.

8 c

Calot's (cystohepatic) triangle is an important anatomical landmark used to identify the cystic artery at cholecystectomy. The triangle is made up of the common hepatic duct, the visceral surface of the right liver and the cystic duct. The cystic artery usually branches from the right hepatic artery inside this triangle.

9 d

The superior mesenteric artery branches from the aorta approximately 1 cm below the origin of the coeliac trunk, at the level of L1. It supplies the derivatives of the midgut, which extend from the major duodenal papilla (the entrance of the bile and main pancreatic ducts) to the proximal two-thirds of the transverse colon.

10 b

The spleen is located beneath the left diaphragm, protected by the ninth to eleventh ribs. It is not normally palpable below the costal margin. Causes of splenomegaly include lymphoma, chronic myeloid leukaemia and sarcoidosis.

11 a

The appendix lies on the posteromedial caecum, lying behind the caecum in 75% of cases. Unlike the caecum it does not have taeniae coli. It is supplied by the appendicular branch of the ileocolic artery.

12 c

Inflammation of the appendix is common and classically presents with initial central umbilical pain with progression to the right iliac fossa. On examination, there is tenderness at McBurney's point, which lies at one-third of the distance from the right anterior superior iliac spine to the umbilicus.

13 a

The superior rectal artery supplies the rectum and anal canal superior to the dentate line. It is the terminal branch of the inferior mesenteric artery, which branches from the aorta at L3.

14 a

The embryological remnant of the umbilical vein is the ligamentum teres, or the round ligament of the liver, which lies on the antero-superior aspect of the liver.

15 c

The islets of Langerhans are responsible for the secretion of hormones from the endocrine pancreas. Glucagon is released from α-cells, insulin from β-cells and somatostatin from δ-cells. Acinar cells secrete enzymes for digestion.

16 d

The hepatic artery and portal vein both supply the liver. Venous drainage occurs via the hepatic vein, which empties directly into the inferior vena cava.

17 e

The sphincter of Oddi controls the flow through the ampulla. The ampulla of Vater marks the anatomical point at which the superior mesenteric artery takes over arterial supply from the coeliac trunk.

18 a

The sigmoid colon connects the descending colon to the rectum and is situated in the left iliac fossa. It is an intraperitoneal part of the gut with a long mesentery.

19 a

The lower oesophageal sphincter (or cardiac sphincter) allows the food bolus to enter the stomach. Gastro-oesophageal reflux disease occurs when the sphincter cannot effectively constrict.

20 c

The caecum is the most proximal part of the large intestine, lying in the right iliac fossa. It acts as a pouch at the start of the ascending colon and overlies both psoas and iliacus muscles.

21 d

Barrett's oesophagus is the process of metaplasia whereby oesophageal squamous epithelium is replaced by columnar cells. Dysplastic change may occur in this area, which can lead to oesophageal carcinoma formation.

22 a

The tail of the pancreas is supplied by the splenic artery, which is one of the three branches of the coeliac trunk, along with the hepatic and left gastric arteries. The pancreatic head is supplied by the superior and inferior pancreaticoduodenal arteries.

23 d

The dentate line is the division of embryological development of the anal canal. Above the dentate line, the canal is formed from columnar epithelium and develops from embryological endoderm. The area of canal below the dentate line develops from endoderm.

24 c

Meckel's diverticulum is the embryological remnant of the vitello-intestinal duct and can be remembered by the '**Rule of 2's**'. It is present in **2**% of the population, although most remain asymptomatic. It is sited **2** feet from the ileocaecal junction, in the distal ileum and is about **2** inches in length. It contains **2** types of ectopic tissue (gastric and pancreatic) and the most common age at presentation is **2** years. Symptoms include pain, bleeding, inflammation and obstruction. Perforation or infection (diverticulitis) of Meckel's diverticulum is clinically indistinguishable from acute appendicitis.

25 a

Five ways in which to differentiate the kidney from the spleen on examination:
- The kidneys are ballotable, the spleen is not.
- The splenic notch on the anterior border can differentiate the two.

- The kidney is resonant (overlying bowel), while the spleen is dull to percussion.
- The spleen enlarges diagonally towards the right lower quadrant.
- The examiner cannot get above the spleen on palpation, while the upper edge of the kidney is palpable.

26 d

In the absence of the Y chromosome the mesonephric (Wolffian) ducts regress. The Müllerian duct differentiates into the female ovaries, uterus and vagina.

27 d

The kidneys are supplied by the paired renal arteries, which branch from the abdominal aorta directly below the superior mesenteric artery. The renal arteries subdivide into five segmental arteries, which further divide into interlobar, arcuate and interlobular arteries.

28 b

The formation of urine begins with glomerular filtration, which occurs between the glomerulus and Bowman's capsule.

29 e

The bladder and ureters are lined with transitional epithelium. Transitional epithelium (or urothelium) allows for distension of the urinary passages and the bladder.

30 c

The kidneys are located between the T12 and L3 vertebrae. The liver displaces the right kidney, therefore it lies slightly lower than the left.

31 c

The prostate receives its blood supply from the internal iliac and internal pudendal arteries.

32 c

The left ureter passes behind the sigmoid colon and travels along the medial border of the psoas muscle. Both the left colic and the gonadal arteries travel over the left ureter. The right ureter is crossed by the right colic, gonadal and ileocolic arteries.

33 d

The pouch of Douglas (or recto-uterine pouch) is a pouch of peritoneum between the bladder and rectum. Because it is the deepest point of the peritoneal cavity, fluid can accumulate here in pathological states (e.g. ascites secondary to malignancy).

34 c

The muscles of the pelvic floor are the levator ani and the coccygeus. The levator ani is comprised of four parts: levator prostatae/vaginae, puborectalis, pubococcygeus and iliococcygeus. Weakness and damage of the pelvic floor from childbirth can result in incontinence and prolapse.

35 b

The natural tone of the internal sphincter and the sympathetic control, causing relaxation of the detrusor, maintain continence until the pressure in the bladder exceeds a critical value. Distension of the bladder wall causes stretch receptors to signal to the cord via pelvic nerves. During micturition, S2–S4 parasympathetic activity causes detrusor muscle contraction and internal sphincter relaxation, facilitating emptying of the bladder. The external sphincter is a striated muscle under somatic control.

36 b

The internal pudendal artery is a branch of the internal iliac and supplies the external genitalia.

37 e

A non-gravid uterus is about 7 cm long and is said to be 'pear-shaped'. At 12 weeks' gestation the uterus can be palpated abdominally and at 20 weeks the fundus reaches the level of the umbilicus.

38 c

The broad ligament houses the Fallopian tubes, the round ligament of the uterus and the uterine artery. The ovaries attach to the broad ligament via the mesovarium.

39 a

As the inferior vena cava (IVC) lies to the right side of the abdomen, the right renal and right gonadal veins drain directly to the IVC. The left gonadal vein, on the other hand drains to the left renal vein and then to the IVC.

40 d

The male urethra is made up of four sections: intramural, prostatic, membranous and spongy urethra, from proximal to distal. The membranous urethra is the narrowest part and therefore also the most vulnerable to trauma on instrumentation.

Theme: Microanatomy of the gastrointestinal tract

1 j

2 a

3 g

4 d

5 e

The parietal cells of the stomach secrete hydrochloric acid in addition to intrinsic factor. Auto-antibodies against these cells, or against intrinsic factor itself, result in pernicious anaemia in which there is a deficiency in vitamin B_{12} absorption. The chief cells secrete pepsin and lipase, involved in the breakdown of protein and fat, respectively. The pancreas has both endocrine and exocrine functions. The islets of Langerhans facilitate the endocrine pancreas: α-cells secrete glucagon, β-cells produce insulin and δ-cells secrete somatostatin. The exocrine acinar cells of the pancreas produce digestive enzymes.

Theme: Anatomy of the gastrointestinal tract

1 j

2 d

3 f

4 k

5 g

The large intestine can roughly be divided into the caecum, colon, rectum and anus. The colon is then subdivided into ascending, transverse and descending parts. The ascending colon travels from the caecum up to the hepatic flexure. It lies retroperitoneal and has no mesentery. The transverse colon lies between the hepatic and splenic flexures and has a mesentery beginning at the inferior edge of the pancreas. The descending colon is retroperitoneal, while the sigmoid colon is intraperitoneal with a long sigmoid mesocolon. The large intestine can be differentiated from the small intestine by various defining features including haustra, taeniae coli and epiploic appendices.

Theme: Anatomy of the hepatobiliary system

1 h

2 f

3 g

4 b

5 d

The breakdown of haemoglobin produces bilirubin. Bilirubin is conjugated by hepatocytes with glucuronic acid. Conjugated bilirubin is water soluble and excreted into the gut with bile. Bile is stored in the gall bladder and passes via the cystic duct, joining with the common hepatic duct to form the common bile duct. The common bile and pancreatic ducts enter the second part of the duodenum at the ampulla of Vater, located at the major duodenal papilla. Obstruction of the common bile duct results in excess conjugated bilirubin in the blood. It enters the urine, resulting in a darkened appearance, while less enters the gut and stool, which subsequently appears paler.

Theme: Vasculature of the gastrointestinal system

1 i

2 e

3 i

4 h

5 c

The three main vessels supplying the gastrointestinal tract are the coeliac trunk and the superior and inferior mesenteric arteries. They supply the derivatives of the foregut, midgut and hindgut, respectively. The coeliac artery divides into its three main branches: left gastric, common hepatic and splenic arteries. The superior mesenteric artery supplies the midgut (from the ampulla of Vater to two-thirds along the transverse colon). Finally, the inferior mesenteric artery branches from the abdominal aorta before it divides into the two common iliac arteries at the level of L4.

Theme: Anatomy of hernias

1 i

2 b

3 e

4 c

5 d

A hernia is an out-pouching of a structure through the wall of the cavity that usually contains it. The most common type of hernia is the inguinal hernia. Inguinal hernias occur superior and medial to the pubic tubercle and are divided into two types: direct and indirect. A direct hernia passes directly through the abdominal wall fascia, while an indirect hernia invaginates through the deep inguinal ring. Femoral hernias are located below and lateral to the pubic tubercle, whereby bowel enters the femoral canal.

Section 4: Cardiorespiratory system

1 c

The bifurcation of the trachea into right and left main bronchi occurs at the level of T4–T5, which also marks the level of the angle of Louis. As the right main bronchus is wider and more vertical than the left, an aspiration pneumonia occurs more commonly on the right.

2 b

The tricuspid valve prevents blood flowing back into the right atrium upon contraction of the right ventricle. Regurgitation through this valve can occur secondary to congenital heart disease, pulmonary hypertension or rheumatic fever. Signs of tricuspid regurgitation include a pansystolic murmur, right ventricular heave and pulsatile hepatomegaly.

3 e

The apex beat is normally located in the fifth intercostal space, mid-clavicular line. It may be displaced infero-laterally (e.g. left ventricular hypertrophy). The nature of the beat is also diagnostically important. It is said to be 'thrusting' in aortic stenosis and has a 'tapping' quality in mitral stenosis.

4 c

The left atrium receives the four pulmonary veins, which carry freshly oxygenated blood from the lungs. The muscular left ventricle then contracts to supply the systemic circulation via the aorta.

5 c

The sinoatrial node is located in the right atrium below the connection of the superior vena cava. The sinoatrial node has the fastest rate of depolarisation and is therefore the primary pacemaker of the heart.

6 b

The oblique fissure is found bilaterally, while the horizontal fissure is only present in the right lung. Fluid can collect in the fissure, which can be identified on a chest radiograph.

7 b

The residual volume is the amount of air remaining in the lungs following a forced expiration. In the average male this volume is approximately 1200 mL. The residual volume prevents the alveoli from collapsing on expiration.

8 b

The posterior interventricular artery is a branch of the right coronary artery that supplies the atrioventricular node in 90% of people. The left coronary artery supplies the atrioventricular node in the remaining 10%.

9 a

As a general rule the superior thyroid artery supplies structures above the vocal cords, while the inferior thyroid artery supplies structures below. Therefore, the inferior thyroid artery supplies the trachea.

10 e

The ventricles are separated by the muscular interventricular septum. A congenital defect in the septum, ventricular septal defect, can present with a pansystolic murmur at birth.

11 d

The right common carotid artery arises from the brachiocephalic trunk, while the left common carotid branches directly from the aortic arch. The left subclavian artery is the third vessel branching from the aortic arch. Bilaterally, the common carotids bifurcate to the internal and external arteries at the level of the upper margin of the thyroid cartilage, at approximately C3–C4. The ophthalmic and inferior hypophyseal arteries are two branches of the internal carotid artery. The ligamentum arteriosum is formed by the closure of the ductus arteriosus at birth. The ductus arteriosus allows blood to shunt from the pulmonary trunk to the descending aorta, thus bypassing the foetal lungs. The right and left laryngeal nerves branch from the vagus; they are anatomically asymmetrical, with the left looped under the ligamentum arteriosum and the right under the right subclavian artery.

12 c

The inferior vena cava passes through the caval opening of the diaphragm at the level of T8, along with branches of the right phrenic nerve. This can be remembered by the following: 'vena cava' has **8** letters and passes through the diaphragm at the level of T**8**.

13 c

Central lines are often used in the intensive care unit setting to measure central venous pressure, to administer drugs and for total parenteral nutrition. It can also be used for dialysis and plasmapheresis. The internal jugular vein is used preferentially to the femoral vein, as infection risk is higher in the groin. The subclavian vein can also be used for catheterisation, although complication rates of pneumothorax are reportedly higher.

14 d

The conducting airways carry inspired gases to the alveoli. As this area does not take part in gaseous exchange, it is known as the anatomical dead space. Oxygen is exchanged for carbon dioxide at the alveoli. An increase in ventilation results in an increase in alveolar oxygen and a decrease in carbon dioxide. The apices of the lungs are ventilated less efficiently than the bases.

15 c

The lung parenchymal tissue and airways are supplied by the bronchial arteries, branches of the thoracic aorta.

16 a

Gases can pass between adjacent alveoli via the pores of Kohn. This allows ventilation to continue in cases of local bronchiole obstruction.

17 e

The vocal cords are formed from the superior and inferior vestibular folds. The space in between the cords is the rima glottidis. The 'true' vocal cords, from the inferior vestibular folds, facilitate vocalisation.

18 e

Type I alveolar cells are squamous cells and create the majority of the alveolar surface. Type II cells produce surfactant, a detergent-like complex that reduces surface tension of the alveoli, thereby increasing compliance.

19 c

The mucosal lining of the respiratory system develops from an outpouching of the foregut endoderm. The muscles and cartilage of the trachea develop from splanchnic mesoderm. The trachea bifurcates early in development and the bronchi continue to branch through to the end of the fourth month. The terminal alveolar sacs form after the seventh month of gestation.

20 c

The neurovascular bundle is located directly below each rib. It consists of anterior and posterior arteries and veins, in addition to the intercostal nerves. Awareness of the position of the neurovascular bundle is important when inserting a chest drain.

21 d

Chest radiographs are one of the most commonly performed investigations in hospital. They are usually taken in the posteroanterior view (i.e. the X-ray source is behind the patient). An anteroposterior film distorts the apparent size of the heart, making it appear larger. The heart is usually less than half the width of the thorax, but can be enlarged in left ventricular hypertrophy and heart failure. The left hilum is higher than the right, although the hila can be pulled up by fibrosis or collapse. The right hemidiaphragm is elevated by the liver and so appears higher than the left.

22 d

Tetralogy of Fallot is the most common cyanotic congenital heart disease. The four cardinal anomalies are an overriding aorta, a large ventricular septal defect, pulmonary stenosis and resultant hypertrophy of the right ventricle.

23 a

The left atrium is the most posterior structure of the heart. The left atrium receives oxygenated blood from the pulmonary veins. Blood passes through the mitral valve and is then, upon contraction of the muscular left ventricle, ejected into the systemic circulation.

24 b

Aortic stenosis results in a hypertrophied left ventricle, as higher pressures are needed to eject blood through the narrowed valve.

25 c

P-waves of the electrocardiogram correspond to atrial contraction, while the QRS waveform is formed by contraction of the ventricles. Absent P-waves may indicate atrial fibrillation, an irregularly irregular rhythm that predisposes patients to the risk of embolic events such as stroke.

26 c

Carcinoma of the lung is divided into small cell and non–small cell carcinoma. There are four distinct non–small cell tumours: adeno-carcinoma and squamous cell, large cell and alveolar cell carcinomas. Adenocarcinoma usually occurs in the periphery of the lung and is proportionally more common in non-smokers.

27 d

Horner's syndrome comprises enophthalmos, anhydrosis, miosis and ptosis. It can result from syringomyelia, demyelination or vascular disease.

28 a

Pancoast's tumour is a lung carcinoma that occurs in the apex. Invasion of the cervical sympathetic plexus results in ipsilateral Horner's syndrome and involvement of the brachial plexus classically leads to shoulder pain and weakness of the upper limb.

29 c

Tuberculosis classically results in patchy/nodular shadowing with signs of fibrosis in the apices of the lungs on a chest X-ray.

30 b

The internal jugular vein is used to assess the jugular venous pressure (JVP). The JVP is the height of the venous pulsation above the sternal angle. This height gives an idea of right atrial pressure. A grossly elevated JVP indicates right ventricular failure.

31 e

Venous return from the systemic circulation enters the right atrium via the superior and inferior venae cavae. The coronary sinus collects the blood from the coronary vessels and also drains into the right atrium.

32 c

Sarcoidosis is a multisystem disorder that can present with pulmonary infiltrates, skin lesions or uveitis. It results from non-caseating granulomas, which consist of epithelioid cells and macrophages. It may be detected incidentally as bilateral hilar lymphadenopathy on a chest X-ray.

33 e

The heart sits within the pericardium, which is a double-layered sac. The outer layer is the fibrous pericardium, which prevents distension of the heart, and the inner layer is the serous pericardium. Between the two layers is a potential space with a thin layer of fluid. The heart and its pericardium lie in the middle mediastinum.

34 b

The perpendicular plate of the ethmoid bone forms the midline nasal septum, while the septal cartilage forms the anterior part.

35 e

The visceral pleura is closely adherent to the lung surface, while the parietal pleura forms an outer layer. The parietal pleura is innervated by intercostal and phrenic nerves, while the visceral pleura is innervated by both anterior and posterior pulmonary plexuses.

36 d

The placenta supplies the foetus with oxygen and nutrients via the umbilical vein. The mother maintains hepatic function and therefore the foetal liver can be bypassed. The ductus venosus shunts blood directly from the umbilical vein to the inferior vena cava, where it mixes with venous blood from the lower parts of the foetus and returns to the right atrium. Blood travels through the foramen ovale to the left atrium. The blood that passes into the right ventricle and to the pulmonary trunk is then shunted through the ductus arteriosus and into the aorta. The aorta connects to the umbilical arteries via the internal iliacs, where deoxygenated blood passes back to the placenta. At birth the umbilical vessels undergo fibrosis. The umbilical arteries become the superior vesical arteries and the medial umbilical ligaments. The umbilical vein forms the ligamentum teres (round ligament of the liver) and the ductus venosus becomes the ligamentum venosum, located on the underside of the liver. In summary:

- ductus venosus → ligamentum venosum
- ductus arteriosus → ligamentum arteriosum
- umbilical vein → ligamentum teres (round ligament of the liver)
- umbilical artery → superior vesical arteries and medial umbilical ligaments.

37 e

The anatomy of the neck is rather complex and so has been anatomically broken down into anterior and posterior triangles. The anterior triangle is bordered by the medial edge of the sternocleidomastoid muscle, the median line of the neck and the mandible, with its apex at the jugular notch of the manubrium. The lateral border of the sternocleidomastoid muscle, the clavicle and the trapezius muscle form the borders of the posterior triangle of the neck. The anterior triangle contains many anatomical structures, including the submental and submandibular lymph nodes, the carotid sheath, the vagus and hypoglossal nerves and the sternothyroid and sternohyoid muscles. The common carotid artery ascends into the anterior triangle, where it bifurcates to form its internal and external branches. The external carotid branches six times before it terminates as the maxillary and superficial temporal arteries. The mnemonic '**A P**olite **O**bese **P**atient **A**sks **S**tudents **T**o **L**ook **F**or **M**any **S**ugary **T**reats!' can be used to remember these vessels:

- **A**scending **P**haryngeal artery

- **O**ccipital artery
- **P**osterior **A**uricular artery
- **S**uperior **T**hyroid artery
- **L**ingual artery
- **F**acial artery
- **M**axillary artery
- **S**uperficial **T**emporal artery.

38 b

Surfactant is a lipoprotein complex that reduces alveolar surface tension, which increases compliance and prevents alveolar collapse on expiration. Because surfactant is produced in the later stages of gestation (>34 weeks), respiratory distress syndrome in premature neonates is common (50% incidence at 32 weeks; over 90% before 28 weeks' gestation). Babies presenting with respiratory distress and cyanosis within 4 hours of birth can be given artificial surfactant down the endotracheal tube, followed by bag ventilation. Corticosteroids administered to the mother a few days before delivery stimulate the synthesis of surfactant and reduce the incidence and mortality of respiratory distress syndrome by up to 40%.

39 e

Pancoast first described apical tumours of the superior pulmonary sulcus in 1932. Invasion of adjacent structures leads to involvement of the sympathetic chain and stellate ganglion, causing Horner's syndrome (anhydrosis, chemosis, miosis and ptosis) on the ipsilateral side. The C8 and T1 nerve roots are frequently involved, causing weakness and wasting of the small muscles of the hand and pain along the distribution of the ulnar nerve. The unique set of symptoms can mimic neurological or musculoskeletal disorders and therefore delayed diagnosis is a major problem.

40 b

Right and left coronary arteries arise from the aorta at the coronary sinus. Maximal flow occurs through the coronary arteries during diastole, as the high pressure in the ventricles during systole cuts off coronary supply. The posterior interventricular branch of the right coronary artery runs in the inferior interventricular groove to supply the atrioventricular node in 90% of people. The coronary vessels drain to the coronary sinus, which runs in the posterior atrioventricular groove, while the anterior cardiac veins can empty directly into the right atrium.

Theme: Cardiac structure and function

1 f

2 c

3 d

4 a

5 e

The right-sided valves are the tricuspid and pulmonary valves, with the aortic and mitral valves on the left. Those separating the atria and ventricles (atrioventricular valves) are the mitral and tricuspid valves. The mitral valve, also known as the bicuspid valve, has two leaflets. The common left-sided systolic murmurs are mitral regurgitation and aortic stenosis: mitral regurgitation is a pansystolic murmur at the apex, while aortic stenosis is an ejection systolic murmur loudest in the aortic region, radiating to the carotids.

Theme: Anatomy of the great vessels

1 a

2 e

3 h

4 f

5 c

The superior and inferior venae cavae drain the systemic circulation to the right side of the heart. Blood is ejected from the right ventricle into the pulmonary artery. The left atrium receives the pulmonary veins, two superior and two inferior; finally, the aorta carries oxygenated blood away from the left ventricle to the systemic circulation.

Theme: Anatomy of the larynx

1 h

2 e

3 d

4 b

5 g

The larynx extends from C4 to C6 and is continuous with the laryngopharynx superiorly and the trachea inferiorly. The U-shaped hyoid bone connects to the thyroid cartilage via the thyrohyoid membrane. The 'shield-like' thyroid cartilage is formed from the fusion of two cartilages and its midline laryngeal prominence gives rise to the 'Adam's apple' in men. The cricoid cartilage lies inferior to the thyroid and is attached by the cricothyroid ligament. The intrinsic muscles of the larynx include the thyroarytenoid, aryepiglottic, interarytenoids and posterior and lateral cricoarytenoids. The recurrent laryngeal nerve supplies all of these muscles. The cricothyroid is an exterior muscle and is supplied by the superior laryngeal nerve.

Theme: Relations of the diaphragm

1 i

2 f

3 b

4 j

5 h

The diaphragm is a muscular dome that separates the thorax from the abdomen. It is supplied via the phrenic nerve from roots C3–C5 (this can be remembered with the mnemonic 'C3, 4, 5 keep the diaphragm alive'). The level at which structures pass through the diaphragm can be remembered by the following:

- 'Vena cava' has **8** letters and passes through at T**8**.
- 'Oesophagus' has **10** letters and passes through at T**10** (along with parts of the vagus nerve, the **10**th cranial nerve).
- 'Thoracic duct' has **12** letters and passes with the aorta at T**12**.

Theme: Anatomy of the airways

1 h

2 c

3 g

4 d

5 a

The trachea arises at the level of C6 and passes down to T4, where it divides into the two main bronchi at the carina. They enter the lung at the hilum and divide into lobar branches. Bronchioles and terminal bronchioles then form the alveoli, where gas exchange occurs. The alveoli have a large surface area and are closely surrounded by a network of pulmonary capillaries, allowing for effective diffusion of oxygen and carbon dioxide. Both lung parenchyma and the airways are supplied by the bronchial arteries from the thoracic arteries.

Index

abdominal aorta
  branches of *(Q)* 55, *(A)* 118
  vessels branching from *(Q)* 42,
    (A) 109
abdominal wall, fascia of *(Q)* 56,
  (A) 119
adrenocorticotrophic
  hormone *(Q)* 18, *(A)* 91
airways
  anatomy of *(Q)* 75, *(A)* 134
  blood supply to *(Q)* 62, *(A)* 123;
    (Q) 75, *(A)* 134
  distal *(Q)* 75, *(A)* 134
alveoli, gas movement
  between *(Q)* 62, *(A)* 123
ampulla of Vater *(Q)* 44, *(A)* 110
  structures entering at *(Q)* 54,
    (A) 117
anal canal, innervation of *(Q)* 46,
  (A) 111
anatomical snuffbox *(Q)* 32, *(A)* 101
angle of Louis *(Q)* 74, *(A)* 133
ankle, dorsiflexion of *(Q)* 27, *(A)* 97;
  (Q) 38, *(A)* 106
antecubital fossa, pulses in *(Q)* 26,
  (A) 97
antidiuretic hormone *(Q)* 11, *(A)* 85
aorta, piercing diaphragm *(Q)* 74,
  (A) 133
aortic arch, vessels arising
  from *(Q)* 35, *(A)* 103; *(Q)* 72,
  (A) 131
aortic valves, stenotic *(Q)* 64, *(A)* 124
apex
  pansystolic murmur at *(Q)* 71,
    (A) 130
  position of *(Q)* 58, *(A)* 120
appendix *(Q)* 42, *(A)* 109

arteries
  in anterior compartment of lower
    leg *(Q)* 26, *(A)* 97
  palpating, *see* pulses
atlas vertebra *(Q)* 31, *(A)* 100
atrial fibrillation *(Q)* 71, *(A)* 130
atrioventricular node, blood supply
  to *(Q)* 59, *(A)* 121
axillary veins *(Q)* 35, *(A)* 103

Babinski reflex *(Q)* 31, *(A)* 100
Baker's cyst *(Q)* 32, *(A)* 100
Barrett's oesophagus *(Q)* 46,
  (A) 111
basal ganglia
  components of *(Q)* 7, *(A)* 82
  and spinal tracts *(Q)* 19, *(A)* 92
biceps-jerk reflex *(Q)* 30, *(A)* 99
bilateral hilar
  lymphadenopathy *(Q)* 67, *(A)* 126
bile, formation of *(Q)* 54, *(A)* 117
bile duct *(Q)* 54, *(A)* 117
bilirubin, formation of *(Q)* 54,
  (A) 117
bitemporal hemianopia
  causes of *(Q)* 7, *(A)* 82
  and lesions *(Q)* 16, *(A)* 89
bladder, lining of *(Q)* 48, *(A)* 112
brachial plexus *(Q)* 31, *(A)* 100
brachiocephalic artery *(Q)* 72,
  (A) 131
branchial cysts *(Q)* 69, *(A)* 127–8

caecum, muscles overlying *(Q)* 45,
  (A) 110
Calot's triangle *(Q)* 41, *(A)* 108–9
cardiac structure and function, *see*
  heart, structure and function

135